Guide to
First Aid
and Medical Terms

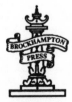

BROCKHAMPTON PRESS
LONDON

This edition published 1996 by Brockhampton Press, a member
of the Hodder Headline PLC Group.

ISBN 1 86019 360 9

Printed and bound in India.

Contents

At the Scene of the Emergency

Before dealing with any patient in need of first aid, it is important to check that you will not actually exacerbate the situation or put yourself at risk. It is vital that you send for specialist help as soon as possible—for this you may be able to use bystanders after instructing them clearly which emergency services you require. You may need to be aware of the safety implications of dealing with a patient in conditions such as heavy traffic or fire, circumstances which will always require increased levels of calm and concentration. You must never be afraid to admit your limitations as a first-aider, and should always be prepared to make way for professionals.

Identifying the Problem: Diagnosis

It can be exceedingly difficult even for doctors to make a diagnosis at times of emergency, without the support of hospital testing facilities. Often it will be impossible for the first-aider to obtain a reliable history from the patient if he or she is unconscious or severely shocked. However, if the first-aider is confident that he can identify life-threatening conditions in the first instance then detailed history-taking is of secondary importance. However, where a patient is unable to give details of events leading up to an accident or emergency, then this information should be sought from any relations or bystanders who might be able to provide useful information. Wherever possible, the first-aider should try to ascertain the patient's name and age and whether or not he has any significant medical problems or is currently taking any medication for a specific condition.

Bites and Stings

When an insect, such as a bee, a wasp or a hornet, stings it injects a tiny amount of venom beneath the skin, causing localized swelling and redness. Although painful, insect stings are rarely serious and the symptoms will begin to subside after 3–4 hours. However, stings can be dangerous, even fatal, if the individual is allergic to the venom or if he has suffered multiple stings. In this case it is essential that the victim receives medical attention immediately.

Insect stings

1 Only honey bees will actually leave their sting embedded in the skin. If the sting is visible, then carefully remove it with the edge of a knife or fingernail. Do not squeeze the sting as this will release more venom.
2 Wash the sting site with soap and water and apply ice wrapped in cloth or a cold compress to the area for up to 30 minutes to reduce the swelling.

Allergic Reaction to an Insect Sting

1 Swelling around the face or on other parts of the body.
2 Difficulty with breathing and swallowing.
3 Weakness and dizziness.
4 Nausea and stomach cramps.
5 Unconsciousness.

To treat an allergic reaction

1 Lie the casualty still and ensure that the stung limb is lower than the level of his heart.
2 Seek emergency medical help immediately.

Animal Bites

Bites which have been caused by an animal or a human should always be referred for medical examination because there is a risk that bacteria on teeth and in saliva will lead to infection.

Bleeding can be quite severe depending upon the type and number of bites, and the first-aider's initial aim should be to control the bleeding.

Treatment for a superficial wound

1 If bleeding is not severe then wash the wound thoroughly with soap and water to try to remove some of the possible contamination.
2 Control bleeding by applying a sterile dressing

or a clean pad and pressing it firmly against
the wound.

3 When bleeding has ceased, cover the wound
with a fresh dressing held in place with
adhesive tape or bandaging.

4 Seek medical examination of the wound. **Do
not** apply medicated ointment to the wound.

Treatment for a severe wound

1 Arrange for the prompt removal of the
casualty to hospital.

2 Control serious bleeding by applying direct
pressure to the wound(s).

3 Cover the wound with a sterile dressing or a
pad of clean cloth.

4 Observe the casualty for signs of shock.

Snakebites

Snakebites are rarely fatal but the venom which is
released in the bite can cause considerable pain to
the victim and may result in illness. It is, therefore,
essential that a snakebite receives medical
examination as soon as possible.

The adder is the only poisonous snake which is
indigenous to Britain—a snake kept in a zoo or
as part of a private collection is likely to be of
foreign origin and it must always be assumed that
such a snake is poisonous.

Treatment for a snakebite

1 Identify the snake if possible and pass this information on to medical staff at the nearest casualty department immediately—this will enable them to identify and prepare the appropriate anti-venom.

2 Before the casualty is transported to hospital, particularly if the journey will take some time, it is important to reduce the amount of venom in the bite wound and inhibit the spread of the venom in the body. Wash the wound with soap and water if possible and cover it with a dressing or a clean cloth. Place a broad bandage just above the site of the wound and fix it firmly but not too tightly in place to make a ligature.

3 Immobilize the affected limb with a splint if possible.

4 Reassure the casualty and observe for signs of shock. Administer mild analgesics such as paracetamol and aspirin if necessary.

6 Arrange for the casualty's immediate removal to hospital.

Bleeding

Blood is the medium in which oxygen is carried to all the living tissues of the body, therefore the loss of any great quantity of blood represents a threat to life itself and should always be treated as a medical emergency. The body has a very sophisticated clotting mechanism which can seal up small lesions quickly and efficiently. Furthermore, a healthy adult may suffer no ill effects after a loss of 850 ml or $1^{1}/_{2}$ pints.

The difficulty in an emergency situation is that it is often impossible to accurately assess the volume of blood which has been lost. It is therefore advisable for the first-aider to take prompt action to stop bleeding wherever possible.

The type of bleeding suffered by a patient will be dependent upon the type of wound sustained. An open wound is one in which there is a visible break in the skin, whereas a closed wound causes the escape of blood from the circulation in to the body tissues. The first kind of bleeding is known as **external** bleeding, and the second is known as **internal** bleeding.

15

Emergency Action for Bleeding

Wherever possible, try to be aware of your own safety. If you have any open wounds, try to ensure that there is a barrier between yourself and the casualty's wound prior to dealing with bleeding.

1 Locate and examine the wound for foreign bodies such as glass. Remove any clothing obstructing your access to the wound. If the wound appears to be free of glass etc., apply pressure directly onto the wound. If the wound is long, or there is a foreign body protruding from it, press down firmly on either side of the wound whilst trying to keep the edges as close together as possible. Apply pressure with a clean pad of material or sterile dressing, but this is not essential and it is important not to waste time searching for one.

2 Elevate the affected part above the level of the patient's heart—you may find it easier to lie the patient down. **Do not** handle a limb you suspect may be fractured other than attempting to stop bleeding.

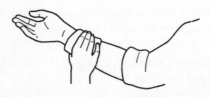

3 Continue to apply pressure for at least 10 minutes. If your original pad or dressing has become saturated, do not remove it. If possible wrap more bandages round it firmly, but not so tightly as to obstruct circulation. Scarves, clean sheets and handkerchiefs etc., make suitable substitutes for bandages.

If the wound contains a foreign body:

1 Make no attempt to pull out the foreign body as this could exacerbate bleeding and shock— it may be acting as a partial 'plug'. However, if it appears loose, it may be possible to flush it out under running water, but do not waste too much time attempting this.

2 Elevate the limb and apply pressure on the edges of the wound. If you have access to sterile gauze pads or any other suitable material, try to build up a platform or ring around the base of the protruding object until it is higher than the object itself. (Leave the object exposed until this is achieved.)

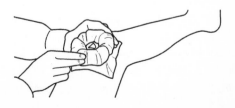

3 Bandage firmly on either side of the wound, but avoiding the wound and the embedded object.

4 Cover the wound loosely with sterile dressings or clean material, elevate the limb and **seek medical help immediately**.

Remember—your priorities are:

1 To control bleeding and prevent shock (see p.94).

2 To prevent or minimize infection.

3 To secure medical help for your patient as quickly as possible.

If despite your best efforts the patient begins to display symptoms of shock, then treat as follows:

1 Identify and treat the cause of shock if possible.

2 Lay the patient flat on the floor as comfortably as possible.

3 Elevate his legs above head height (unless you suspect a fracture).

4 Loosen or remove any restrictive articles of clothing.

5 Keep the patient warm by covering with blankets, rugs or coats, but do not apply a direct heat source such as a hot water bottle.

6 Keep a check on the patient's vital signs— pulse and respiration, and his level of

consciousness. Be ready to resus-citate if
necessary (see ABC of Resuscitation on p.68).

Internal Bleeding

Internal bleeding may result from injury such as
bone fracture or severe bruising, but it can also
occur spontaneously as a result of stomach ulcer
or vaginal bleeding or several other medical
emergencies. In the absence of any visible blood,
the diagnosis is often a hard one to make, but signs
and symptoms of shock (see p.96) will emerge if
internal bleeding is significant. Sometimes there
will be blood present at body orifices, and there
may be bruising. Always treat for shock and
summon medical help immediately.

Nosebleeds

Nosebleeds are rarely serious and most commonly
occur either after a blow to the nose, during an
infection such as the common cold, or as a
consequence of picking or blowing the nose.
Occasionally, frequent nosebleeds may be a result
of high blood pressure, or a sign of a weak blood
vessel inside the nose which ruptures
spontaneously from time to time. Normally,
nosebleeds are simply inconvenient and
unpleasant, but occasionally they can be
dangerous if bleeding is prolonged as the casualty

can suffer considerable blood loss perhaps
resulting in shock. If the blood coming from the
nose appears thin and watery, summon medical
help immediately as this may indicate leakage of
fluid from around the brain as a result of head or
facial injury.

To Treat a Nosebleed

1 Seat the patient comfortably with his head
  forward. Do not tip the head back in an
  attempt to stop bleeding, as the patient will be
  forced to swallow the blood as it trickles down
  the back of his throat which may cause
  vomiting.

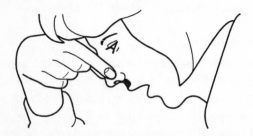

2 Pinch the patient's nose just beneath the bridge
  and ask her to breathe through the mouth.
3 Ask her not to speak, sniff or swallow if
  possible as this may hinder clots from forming.
4 Apply pressure for a full 10 minutes in the first
  instance. If bleeding persists, apply a further

10 minutes' pressure. If bleeding has not ceased completely within 30 minutes, consult a doctor immediately or take the patient to the nearest accident and emergency unit. The patient should remain in the treatment position while travelling.

5 If bleeding stops, clean gently around the nose with cotton wool or a swab soaked in warm water. Ask the patient not to blow her nose for at least 4 hours and to rest quietly to avoid dislodging the clot.

Breathing Difficulties

Asthma

Asthma is an increasingly common respiratory disorder which can be triggered by allergy, exertion, cigarette smoke, respiratory infection, or by emotional factors. The patient will experience increasing tightness in the chest and difficulty in breathing as the air passages constrict. Breathing is characterized by wheezing, which may be audible as a whistling sound particularly when the patient breathes out. Most asthma sufferers cope well with the problem, and will usually be aware of the onset of an attack and take appropriate medication, usually in the form of inhalers. However, if it is the patient's first attack and he does not have medication, or if medication has been taken but without any response, it is essential that medical help is summoned immediately as asthma can be fatal.

Symptoms of an asthmatic attack

1 Difficulty in breathing, anxiety and difficulty in speaking.

2 Blueish appearance to the face, especially around the lips.

To treat an attack of asthma

1 Sit the patient at a table and encourage him to lean forward with his arms resting on the top of a table.

2 Ensure the room has an adequate supply of fresh air. Open a window, but not if the weather is cold.

3 Reassure the patient and encourage him to take his medication.

4 If there has been no response to the inhaler within 10–15 minutes, or if the patient becomes drowsy or begins to go blue around the lips, telephone for an ambulance immediately.

Croup

Croup is a breathing disorder of very young children caused by inflammation of the trachea (windpipe) and larynx. It is characterized by a barking cough, perhaps accompanied by a wheezing or whistling sound (known as **stridor**) and in severe cases the child may appear blue. It frequently occurs at night and can be very alarming, but an attack almost always resolves itself without further problems. Recovery can be quickened by:

1 Taking the child into a steam-filled room, such as a bathroom with the hot tap running in the bath.
2 Keeping the atmosphere in the child's bedroom humid.

It is advisable to call your doctor as the condition can recur after the initial attack has subsided.

If the child is sitting bolt upright or has a high temperature, this may indicate a more serious condition known as **epiglottitis** which requires immediate medical attention.

Hyperventilation

Hyperventilation occurs when an individual experiences an emotional fright, upset or stress. It is characterized by a shallow, rapid breathing pattern, whereby too much carbon dioxide is removed from the body. This will cause feelings of dizziness and tingling, and may cause the individual to panic. Adequate carbon dioxide levels can be restored and the symptoms controlled by encouraging the individual to breath into a paper bag held over his nose and mouth for up to 4 minutes.

Burns and Scalds

Burns are sustained in a number of ways—most commonly from dry heat, friction or corrosive chemicals, whilst scalds are caused by liquids and vapours. Although heat accounts for most burns and scalds, it is important to remember that contact with extreme cold can also burn, as can radiation.

At the scene of the burns incident:

1 Make sure you do not put yourself in danger from the presence of fire, electrical hazards, etc.
2 Where possible, stop the burning of affected tissues by rapid cooling. The most effective way of doing this is to place the affected limb or part under cold running water **for at least 10 minutes**. This will help to minimize tissue damage, swelling, shock and pain.

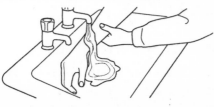

3 If removing the patient to hospital, turn off the water and cover the wound. A **non-stick** sterile dressing is preferable, but if not available, a clean handkerchief, pillowcase or sheet will do. Burns are highly vulnerable to infection, so it is important not to leave a wound exposed to the atmosphere for any length of time.

4 Keep the patient as calm as possible and observe for signs of shock (see p.96). Always obtain medical help quickly for all but the most minor of burns.

Never use an adhesive dressing on a burn.

Never apply creams, ointments, sprays, butter or indeed anything else to a burn—these will have to be removed and will cause additional pain and distress to the sufferer.

Never prick or burst any blister which appears on a burn—these are nature's defence against infection.

Never try to remove anything sticking to a burn—in fact try not to touch or interfere with the affected area at all.

Burns to the Mouth and Throat

Burns on the face and mouth are extremely serious as they can cause rapid swelling of the airways. Summon medical help immediately and be

prepared to resuscitate. Inform the ambulance
service that you suspect burns of the airway.

Electrical burns

Burns may be caused by an electrical current
passing into the body. Although most damage is
done at the points of entry and exit, occasionally
tracks of damage are caused internally. Severe
electric shock may cause cardiac arrest—if the
victim is unconscious, disregard any burns
initially and give priority to the ABC of
Resuscitation (see p.70).

If the source of electricity is Low Voltage,
such as domestic supply it is essential to isolate
the casualty from the current either by
disconnecting the power or using wood or plastic
to separate the victim from the appliance.
Alternatively wrench the cable from the plug or
grab the victims clothing and pull her free. **Do
not come into contact with the victim's skin**.

Thereafter
1 Treat the site of injury as for any other burn.
2 Observe and treat the victim for shock and
   summon an ambulance.

Chemical burns

Chemicals which cause severe burns are normally
found in industry, but some paint strippers and

other domestic chemicals can also inflict similar burns. Try to find out what the substance was in order to inform the doctor, and summon medical help immediately. In the meantime:

1 Flood the burnt area with copious amounts of running water. Protect yourself with rubber gloves.
2 Remove any clothing which is likely to be contaminated with the chemical.
3 Get the casualty to hospital as quickly as possible.

Chemical Burns to the Eyes

If the eyes are affected, it is essential to pour as much water into them as possible. This will obviously need to be done as gently as possible, and as the eyes will probably be tightly shut in pain, it may be necessary to prise them open firmly. Chemical burns to the eyes can cause lasting damage and even blindness, therefore it is essential to seek hospital treatment without delay.

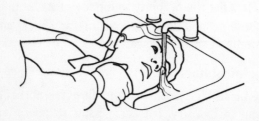

Choking

Normally when we swallow, a flap of cartilage known as the epiglottis moves downwards to stop food being taken into the trachea or windpipe. Where this fails to happen, food becomes stuck in the airway and choking is said to have occurred. Sometimes, the victim may appear to vomit or cough up the foreign body, but occasionally this fails to happen and the patient may be unable to breathe either partially or completely. Where a choking victim is unable to breathe, action must be taken immediately, as brain damage will occur within three or four minutes of its being starved of oxygen. Choking is a common cause of accidental death amongst children.

How to Recognize a Choking Attack

1 The victim will probably clutch at his or her throat and be unable to speak.

2 The victim will probably become acutely distressed and panicky.

3 Inability to breathe will probably result in fairly rapid loss of consciousness.

Emergency Action for a Choking Attack in an Adult

1 Lean the victim forwards and give her 5 hard slaps on the back between the shoulder blades.

2 If this is unsuccessful, then abdominal thrusts can be performed from behind a patient who is either standing or sitting. For this, pass your hands around the patient and interlock your hands together just above the navel in the region of the diaphragm and pull sharply inwards and upwards.

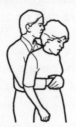 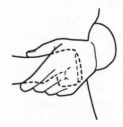

3 If the casualty is unconscious, kneel astride her on the floor and perform similar abdominal thrusts with the heel of the hand (one hand positioned on top of the other) just below the rib-cage

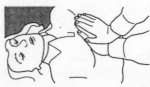

4 If you have tried abdominal thrusts six times without response, telephone 999 for an ambulance and begin resuscitation immediately (see p. 70).

Emergency Action for a Choking Child

1 Lay the child across your lap with its head down. Slap firmly between the shoulder blades five times .
2 Should this be unsuccessful, turn him over so he faces you on your lap. Support the back of and give him five firm upward thrusts with one hand above his navel.
3 Should this fail to dislodge the foreign body, then try steps 1 and 2 again. If the child becomes unconscious, then call an ambulance immediately and begin resuscitation (see p.70).

Emergency Action for a Choking Baby

Abdominal thrusts should **never** be used on a child younger than 1 year.
1 Straddle the baby face down along your arm suuporting her head and give her five firm slaps between the shoulders.
2 If choking continues, turn the baby over, still supporting the back of her head. Place two fingertips between the navel and the breastbone. Press forward and downward in

quick movements and repeat the movement up to four times if necessary.

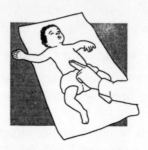

3 If the infant loses consciousness, summon medical help immediately and begin resuscitation.

Remember

Never poke your fingers down a choking victim's throat in an attempt to find the obstructing object—you will only push it in further and make it more difficult to dislodge. If the object appears in or at the victim's mouth, then you may remove it gently.

Drowning

Drowning is one of the most common causes of accidental death, especially in children, but is often quite hard to recognize in the initial stages. It may be very hard for a person drowning to summon the energy to shout, therefore the sight of a swimmer waving should always be treated with suspicion. The victim will attempt to hold his breath for as long as possible, but will eventually be forced to take a breath, permitting water to enter the airway. The muscles in the throat will respond by going into spasm which will then restrict breathing. The patient will quickly lapse into unconsciousness as the oxygen supply to the brain is cut off.

The brain will sustain permanent damage after it has been deprived of oxygen for just 3–4 minutes, unless the water is very cold. Under these circumstances, the brain may require less oxygen, and may survive unharmed for up to 30 minutes or more, particularly in the case of children. Therefore, it is always worth resuscitating a victim who has been pulled from cold water, even if you suspect he has been submerged for longer than 4 minutes.

Rescue and Treatment of a Drowning Victim

1 **Do not risk your own safety**. Try to reach the victim from land by extending a pole or a rope. **Do not** attempt to swim or wade to him through a strong current or deep, cold water as you may find yourself quickly overcome.

2 If you are carrying the victim to safety try to ensure that you have a floating object, such as a board or a lifebelt, that he can grab hold of; in his panic he may grab you and thus make it more difficult for you to keep afloat. Keep his head tilted below the level of his body to allow as much water to drain naturally as possible. Similarly, when laying the victim down, try to do so on a slope with his head down-most.

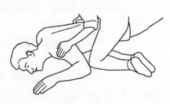

3 Check the airway for signs of obstruction with weeds or other debris, and clear by using finger sweeps, except in very small children. **Do not** use abdominal thrusts as this may cause stomach contents to be inhaled.

4 If the victim still has a carotid pulse but is failing to breathe, then begin mouth-to-mouth ventilation straight away (see p.70).

5 If there is no carotid pulse or breathing, then send someone for an ambulance and give full cardio-pulmonary resuscitation (see p.73).

6 Even though your patient appears to have made a full recovery, always send him to hospital for observation as serious breathing difficulties may recur some hours after the accident. Whilst awaiting the arrival of the emergency services, keep the patient as warm as possible, as he may be suffering from hypothermia.

Fainting and Fits

Epilepsy

Epilepsy is a common condition in which the sufferer experiences a fit or seizure in response to sudden disruption of normal electrical activity in the brain. In an attack, the casualty may suddenly fall to the ground unconscious. For a few seconds, his muscles may stiffen and breathing will stop. This is known as the **tonic** phase, and is succeeded by the **clonic** phase, in which the whole body jerks violently, and breathing recommences noisily through clenched teeth. Normally, the jerking will cease and the muscles relax within about a minute. Breathing will become normal again, but the patient may remain unconscious for a few more minutes.

Although an epileptic fit can be frightening to witness, they rarely cause the sufferer any lasting harm, unless they have injured themselves during the fall or the clonic phase.

How to Help During an Epileptic Fit

1 Move furniture and other objects to clear a

space around the patient, and if possible
position him on his back before the jerking
begins.

2 Loosen tight clothing, but do not attempt to
restrain the patient or put anything in his
mouth during the attack.

3 When the convulsion has subsided, place the
patient in the recovery position (see p.79) and
remain with him until he has made a complete
recovery.

4 Examine the patient for signs of injury such as
cuts or fractures. When he is fit to move,
ensure that he gets home safely and informs
his doctor, especially if this is the first attack.

5 If the patient does not regain consciousness
within 15 minutes, or has repeated convulsions
then call an ambulance.

Fainting

Fainting is a temporary loss of consciousness
occasioned by a reduced blood supply to the brain.
This may be caused by an emotional shock, fear,
pain or inadequate food intake over a period of
time. More usually, however, people faint after
long spells of inactivity, particularly in warm,
airless conditions, during which blood will tend to
pool in the lower part of the body, thereby
reducing the amount available to the brain.

Treatment of fainting:

1 Lie the casualty down on the floor and raise his legs above the level of his head.

2 Open the windows and wait for the casualty to regain consciousness—usually within a few minutes.

3 If the patient recovers, but continues to feel faint, ask him to sit with his head down between his knees.

4 If the casualty does not regain consciousness quickly, place him in the recovery position (see p.79), check pulse and respiration and call for an ambulance. Be prepared to resuscitate if necessary.

Febrile Convulsion

Febrile convulsions are caused by overheating and are most common in the under 2's. There is usually a history of fever and illness such as throat infection, which is often exacerbated by wrapping the child too warmly in bed. Typically, the child's skin will be flushed and hot, and the convulsion is characterized by arching of the back and violent muscle-twitching. The fists may be clenched and the eyes rolled upwards, and the breath is often held.

Treatment of a febrile convulsion is aimed at reducing the child's body temperature.

1 Remove the child's blankets and clothing.

2 Sponge the child with a sponge or flannel soaked in tepid water starting from the head and working downwards.

3 Keep the airway open by placing the child in the recovery position (see p.79).

4 Pad around the child with soft pillows to prevent him from hurting himself during a convulsion.

5 Call the doctor.

Foreign Bodies

Foreign Body in the Nose

A foreign body that is lodged in the nose should always receive medical attention. Attempts to remove the object, particularly if it is sharp, may cause damage to the tissue.

Signs and symptoms

1 The casualty will appear to have some difficulty in breathing through the nose.
2 Bleeding or discharge from one or both nostrils will be apparent.
3 The nose may be swollen.

Treatment

1 Advise the patient to breathe through his mouth.
2 Reassure him and arrange for him to receive medical attention as soon as possible.

Foreign Body in the Ear

As with foreign bodies in the nose, this type of injury is often sustained by young children. In most cases no attempt should be made to remove the foreign body as this may cause serious injury to the delicate ear drum; it is essential that the casualty receives medical attention as soon as possible.

Signs and symptoms

1 The patient may complain of impaired hearing in the affected ear.
2 The patient will complain of pain or discomfort in the ear.

Foreign Body in the Eye

Foreign bodies in the eye are fairly common. Eyelashes or small particles of dust, sand or grit often become lodged underneath the eyelid or stuck to the surface of the eyeball. While these can cause the casualty discomfort and the eye tissue to become inflamed, they are usually quite easily removed. However, if a foreign body is embedded in the eyeball or is on the iris, then no attempt should be made to remove it; in such cases the casualty should always receive medical treatment.

Signs and symptoms

1 The casualty will complain of discomfort and will probably attempt to rub the unaffected eye.
2 The affected eye will appear red and inflamed and will water.

3 The patient may complain that his vision is impaired.

Treatment

1 Discourage the patient from rubbing his eye and reassure him.

2 If possible, sit the casualty in a chair and ask him to lean his head back.

3 Examine the casualty's eye, supporting his chin with one hand and using the other hand (index finger and thumb) to open the eye wide by stretching the upper and lower lid. If you ask the casualty to move his eyeball up and down, and from left to right you will be able to examine the eyeball more effectively.

4 If you can locate the foreign body try to remove it by washing it out with distilled water or fresh tap water if this is not available. Lean the head over on the affected side so that the water runs away down the cheek. If water is not readily accessible then try to use a moistened swab, such as the corner of a damp, clean handkerchief.

5 If the foreign body is embedded on the iris (the coloured area of the eye) or cannot be removed using steps 1–4, then the casualty should receive medical attention. Try to cover the eye with a sterile dressing (ideally and eye pad)

and secure it in place, ensuring that there is not
too much pressure applied to the eyeball
6 Arrange for the casualty to be removed to
hospital.

Ingested Foreign Bodies

A foreign body which has been swallowed may, if
sharp, cause choking or result in damage being
caused to the gastro-intestinal tract. Never attempt
to make the casualty vomit as a method of
removing the object, this will inevitably result in
much greater damage and distress.

If the casualty has swallowed a foreign object
then it is important to ascertain precisely what the
object and remove the casualty to hospital as
soon as possible. Do not allow the patient to take
anything by mouth, reassure him and observe for
signs of discomfort.

Fractures

A fracture is a crack or break in a bone. It takes a considerable degree of force to break bones as they are not simply brittle sticks but living tissues supporting the body. However, the bones of the elderly or those affected by disease may become more brittle and vulnerable, whilst those of children may be more likely to split under force as they are more supple. Bones are supplied with a rich network of nerves and blood vessels, which accounts for the amount of pain and swelling experienced when a fracture is sustained.

Types of Fracture

1 Simple fracture: A clean break in a bone.
2 Compound fracture: A break in which the broken bone pierces the skin or is accompanied by a wound. In a compound fracture, the bone is exposed to contamination by infection from the air.
3 Comminuted fracture: The bone is shattered into several fragments at the site of the break.
4 Greenstick fracture: Most commonly experienced by children. This type of fracture

will show up on an X-ray as an incomplete
break or split in a bone.

5 Pathological fracture: The bone may break
spontaneously where affected by disease or
some other weakening factor such as a cyst.

Signs and Symptoms of Fracture

1 The patient may report having heard or felt a
snap, although this can be caused by injuries
other than fracture.

2 The patient will often experience severe pain
which is worsened by attempts to move the
limb.

3 The patient will be unable to move the limb
normally as a result of the pain and the
instability of the broken bone.

4 Bleeding from the damaged bone and
surrounding tissues will quickly result in
swelling. Some time later, bruising will
probably occur, again as a result of
haemorrhage within the tissues.

5 The limb may be misshapen or deformed as a
result of the break, or thrown into an unnatural
position.

How to help a fracture victim

1 With the exception of suspected fractures to
small bones in the upper limbs, it is best not to

move the casualty, especially if you suspect his spine may be fractured.

2 Steady the broken limb by holding it gently but firmly above and below the fracture site, but do not attempt to straighten it.

3 Dial 999 for an ambulance at your earliest possible opportunity.

4 It may be possible to immobilize the injured part without moving it unduly. For example, it may be possible to support a broken leg between two cushions or folded clothing, but do not attempt this if it involves moving the limb or altering its position. It is always a good idea to immobilize a broken arm against the body using a sling.

5 If it looks as if help may be some time in arriving, a broken leg may be gently secured to the sound leg with bandages. However, do not persist with this if it seems to be causing additional pain or distress.

6 Reassure the patient and observe for shock (see p.96)

7 Keep the patient warm, but do not give him anything to eat or drink, as he may require a general anaesthetic on admission to hospital.

Open Fractures

Open fractures (i.e. those in which the broken

bone is exposed to the air through a wound in the skin) should be treated in much the same way as closed fractures. The main problem is that as the wound is open, it is more prone to infection and there may be considerable blood loss. As with any fracture, it is essential to arrange for early removal of the casualty to hospital. Whilst waiting for the ambulance to arrive, proceed as follows:

1 Support the wound in the same way as you would with a closed fracture.
2 Gently cover the wound with a sterile dressing or clean pad of material.
3 Place more padding such as cotton wool around the pad and build it high enough to prevent pressure on any protruding bone (see illustration on p.17).
4 Bandage the padding gently but firmly in place. Take care not to bandage it so tightly that it impedes circulation or causes the patient further pain.
5 If possible elevate and immobilize the limb.
6 Reassure the patient and observe for shock (see p.96).

Facial fractures

Broken noses, cheekbones and jaws are among the most common injuries to the face. The main problems with injuries of this type is that the airway may become blocked by swelling or bleeding, or perhaps by teeth which have been dislodged. Bear in mind that the blow which caused the most obvious injury may also have caused damage to the skull, the neck or even the brain.

Injuries/Fractures of the Nose and Cheekbones

These injuries frequently occur as a result of fighting and can cause considerable discomfort as swelling progresses. The aim of the first-aider is to reduce the swelling and to have the patient examined in hospital as soon as possible. Treat swelling as follows:

1 Apply a cold compress. (A flannel or large handkerchief soaked in cold water then frequently refreshed will suit this purpose.)
2 Take or send the patient to hospital.

Fracture of the Lower Jaw

This injury is usually caused by direct force to the jaw, either by a blow or a heavy fall. The pain can be excruciating, and is often exacerbated by movement of the jaw which is often hard to avoid. Fast removal of the patient to hospital is vital, but in the meantime you can make her more comfortable.

1 Encourage her to sit upright with her head
  tilted forward. This will encourage blood and
  saliva to drain from the mouth rather than
  necessitating swallowing.

2 Give the patient a soft pad
  and allow her to hold it in
  place against the painful
  jaw to support it.
  Encourage her to keep the
  jaw supported or tie a
  narrow bandage around the head until she
  reaches the hospital.

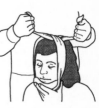

If the Facial Injury Victim is Unconscious

1 Check frequently that the airway is clear.
2 Place her in the recovery position (see p.79).
3 Call an ambulance immediately.
4 If a fractured jaw is suspected, slip a pad of
  soft material under the head in order to prevent
  its weight resting on and further damaging the
  jaw.

  **Remember that an injury above chest level
should be treated as a suspected Spinal Injury**.

Fractures of the Upper Limb

The term 'upper limb' includes not only the arm
but also the shoulder and the collar bone. If the
patient can walk without too much distress, then it

may be unnecessary to call an ambulance, although hospital treatment is essential.

Fracture of the Collar-bone

The collar-bone is situated at the base of the neck and supplies the arm's support between the breastbone and the shoulder-blade. Fractures are usually a result of indirect force, such as an outstretched hand during a fall transmitting the force up to the collar-bone. The patient will undoubtedly experience pain at the injury site, and will frequently attempt to relieve this by tilting the head to one side. If a fractured collar-bone is suspected:

1 Immobilize the arm on the injured side by sitting the patient down and placing the arm on the affected side across her chest with her fingertips resting lightly on the opposite shoulder.

2 Place some padding between the injured limb and the casualty's chest. Support the arm in this position in an elevation sling across the shoulder (see p.63).

3 Give the arm further support if possible by adding an additional broadfold bandage around the chest.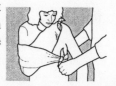

4 Take the patient to hospital.

Dislocation of the Shoulder

Dislocation of the shoulder is most commonly caused by a fall. In dislocation, the ball-type shoulder joint is wrenched out of its socket causing extreme pain, especially upon movement. The first-aider's main aim is to reduce the pain by immobilizing the joint until the casualty can be taken to hospital—**do not** attempt to relocate the joint. Seat the patient then:

1 Gently position the affected arm across the chest and apply an arm sling (see p.62).
2 Slip some padding behind the sling to give further support on the affected side. Check that the sling is not too tight by feeling for the pulse or numbness in the fingers
3 Arrange for the patient to be taken to hospital.

Fracture of the Upper Arm

Fractures of the long bone (humerus) in the upper arm occur most commonly as a result of a fall, although can occasionally result from a direct blow. There will commonly be extreme pain accompanied by bruising and/or swelling at the site of the fracture. As with other arm injuries, hospital treatment is called for but first

1 Seat the patient.
2 Apply a sling and broad fold bandage (see p.60).

Fractures around the Elbow

These are fairly common and are characterized by pain and swelling, which will be worsened by movement. With this type of fracture, there is increased danger of damage to surrounding nerves and blood vessels, therefore it is best to call an ambulance rather than attempting to take the patient to hospital on your own. If the elbow can still be bent, then use a sling as previously described for other arm injuries. If the arm cannot be bent:

1 Immobilize the arm by placing some padding between the arm and the trunk, then securing the arm against the body with large, broad bandages.

2 Check the patient's wrist pulse every 10 minutes. If pulse is absent loosen the bandaging and ask the patient to reposition his arm if possible until pulse returns. Call an ambulance.

Fractures of the Hip and Leg

When attending a casualty with a fracture of the leg or hip it is important that an ambulance is summoned as soon as possible. The casualty should not be moved unless medical assistance cannot be summoned or you have to remove him from a situation of potential danger. Fractures of

the hip and thigh bone are often characterized by
shortening and outward rotation of the injured
limb. Should you need to move the patient:

1 Gently lay the casualty on his back, supporting
the injured limb with your hand, and make him
as comfortable as possible.

2 Place plenty of soft padding between the legs,
from the groin to the ankle. If long, straight
boards or branches are available then prepare
to use these as splints. One splint should be
long enough to reach from the groin to the
ankle and the other from the armpit to the
ankle. Pad the shorter splint, lay it gently
between the legs and gently bring the sound
limb alongside the fractured leg.

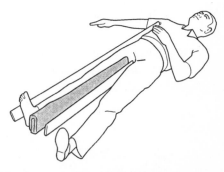

3 Place padding from the casualty's armpit to the
ankle of the injured leg and then bandage as
illustrated, avoiding the fracture site and

ensuring that the knots are tied over the splint. Apply more padding between his arm and the outer surface of the long splint.

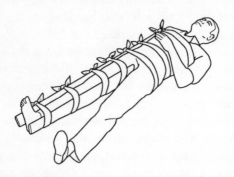

4 If splints are not available then gently place thick padding between the casualty's legs and bandage the legs together, avoiding the fracture site and ensuring that knots are tied over the padding. Minimize movement and discomfort by using a thin stick to push the bandages underneath the legs.

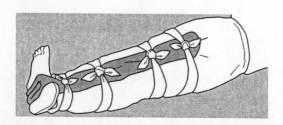

6 Once the limbs are immobilized, if possible raise them a little to reduce the swelling. Check the ankles for signs of a pulse and the toes for numbness; loosen the bandages a little if necessary.

7 Observe the casualty for shock (see p.96) and ensure that he is kept warm and as comfortable as possible.

Fractures of the Lower Leg

Fractures to the bones of the lower leg are frequently characterized by an open fracture, whereby the broken bone protrudes throught the skin. It is, therefore, important to gently cover the wound with the cleanest dressing or material available and summon medical assistance as soon as possible. You should never attempt to straighten the fractured bone or to move the injured limb unnecessarily. To immobilize the leg you should:

1 Gently lie the casualty on his back and ensure that he is as comfortable as possible.

2 Use two splints which both extend from well above the knee to below the ankle. Place the splints along the inner and outer side of the fractured leg, applying padding in between the splints and the leg on both sides.

3 Tie the splints to the leg with bandages or material in up to four places, always avoiding

the site of the fracture. Ensure that the knots are tied over the splint.

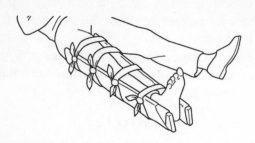

4 If splints are not available gently try to straighten the knee of the injured leg if it is bent. Place padding between the legs and move the sound leg alongside the injured limb.

5 Tie the feet using a figure of 8 bandage, then tie a bandage around the knee. Apply 2–3 more bandages, avoiding the fracture site and ensuring that the knots are tied on the uninjured side.

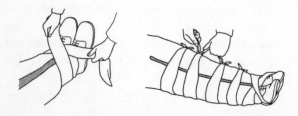

Fracture of the Spine

Suspected fracture of the spine should always be
treated as a serious injury and medical help should
be sought urgently. Fracture to the vertebrae, the
small bones which make up the spine, may be
complicated by the risk of damage to the spinal
cord which is enclosed within the spinal column.
The spinal cord is composed of nerve tissue which
transmits impulses from the brain which control
many of the functions of the body. Any damage to
the spinal cord could, thus, result in temporary or
permanent paralysis in parts of the body,
depending on where the injury occurs. It is
therefore essential that the casualty is
immobilized as far as possible to minimize the
risk of damage.

Symptoms of spinal injury

1 The victim may complain of severe pain in the
   back.
2 Lack of control over movement in the limbs.
3 Loss of sensation in the limbs, even when
   touched gently.

Treatment of spinal injury

When attending a casualty with a back injury,
where the precise nature of the injury is unclear,
always treat it as a fracture.

1 Arrange for the casualty to be removed to hospital, by ambulance, as soon as possible.

2 Support the casualty by gently steadying him head with your hand and placing rolled up clothing, blankets and towels around the trunk of his body. Secure these in place with bricks, stones or heavy bags. Cover the casualty with a blanket and keep as comfortable as possible.

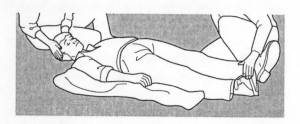

3 If the victim is in imminent danger and has to be moved immediately, then he must be supported at the head and neck, the shoulders, the waist and the legs to ensure that the head, neck and torso are in alignment.

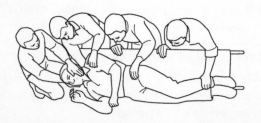

4 The casualty should always be carried any distance on a rigid stretcher or board with the limbs gently supported.

Dislocated Bones

Articulating joints, such as the shoulder or hip, are held together by strong strips of tissue called ligaments. The ligaments generally hold the joint in the correct position and ensure its correct movement, but occasionally violent movement or injury can tear the ligament thus permitting dislocation or displacement of the bone. Contrary to popular belief, **no attempt** should be made to replace the joint, as this can result in further injury. The best course of action is to treat the dislocation as a fracture and ensure the swift removal of the patient to hospital for treatment.

Bandages and Slings

A basic triangular bandage can be adapted for use as a sling or for using as a broad or narrow bandage or a ring pad. These can be made by cutting a piece of material (approximately 1 metre by 1 metre) in half diagonally.

Broad bandage

Broad bandages can be used for immobilizing limbs before transporting a casualty.

Using the triangular bandage, fold in the point towards the base of the bandage and then fold in half again.

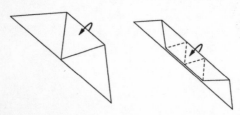

Narrow bandage

A narrow bandage can be used for securing a dressing in place, making a ring pad and for fixing a figure of eight bandage.

Using a triangular bandage make a broad bandage as shown above and then simply fold in half again.

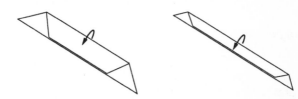

Ring pad

When used on a complicated fracture where the bone is protruding through the skin or on a wound where a foreign body is present, a ring pad can be used to provide protection around the wound and prevent dressings from creating too much pressure.

1 Make a narrow bandage as hown above and wrap it once around the fingers of one hand to make a loop.

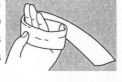

2 Take hold of the other end of the bandage and wind it around the loop, pulling it tight.

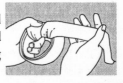

3 Continue to firmly wind the bandage around the loop until the bandage has been used and tuck in the end.

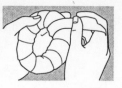

Arm sling

An arm sling should provide support for the forearm, elbow and wrist. It should be applied so that the hand is slightly higher than the elbow and the fingertips are exposed. Always apply a sling with the casualty standing or sitting down and work from the injured side to provide more support.

1 Support the arm across the chest, ensuring that the hand is slightly higher than the elbow. Take a triangular bandage and slide one end underneath the forearm until the point of the bandage reaches well below the elbow.

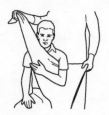

2 Take the upper end of the sling, place it around the shoulder on the uninjured side, then take it around the back of the neck and then to the front on the injured side.

3 Take the lower end of the sling and fold it over the forearm and then tie it off in the hollow above the collar-bone.

4 Take the point of the bandage and fold it forward onto the front, fixing it with a safety pin and ensuring that the casualty's fingertips are not covered.

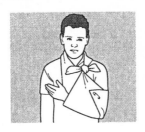

Elevation sling

An elevation sling should be used to support an injury to the shoulder or where a hand wound is bleeding. The aim is to raise and support the forearm and the hand.

1 Gently place the forearm on the injured side across the chest so that the fingertips are level with the opposite shoulder. Ask the casualty to support the limb if possible.

2 Place the base of a triangular bandage over the raised forearm and hand so that the upper end

sits on the shoulder on the uninjured side and the point reaches beyond the tip of the elbow.

3 Gently slide the base of the bandage underneath the elbow, forearm and hand.

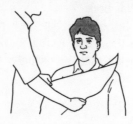

4 Take the lower end of the sling and place it around the casualty's back and across to the shoulder on the uninjured side. Tie it off in the hollow of the collar-bone and adjust if necessary.

5 Take the point of the sling and tuck it between the forearm and the front of the sling. This will leave a fold of material which can be pinned back against the arm.

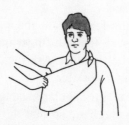

Remember—when applying bandages and slings ensure that the casualty's circulation is not affected. If so then adjust the bandage or reposition the sling until circulation has improved.

Heart Attack and Cardiac Arrest

A heart attack is said to have occurred when a clot of blood suddenly blocks a coronary artery, one of the main blood vessels to the heart muscle, the **myocardium.** When this happens, the affected part of muscle will die due to the resulting lack of oxygen causing the patient severe, gripping chest pain. Sometimes, the patient may have a history of **angina pectoris,** a condition in which the coronary arteries are narrowed due to the build-up of fatty deposits on the inside walls. This restricts the blood flow to the myocardium and causes severe crushing pain in the chest, not unlike that of a heart attack. Therefore, it is sometimes very difficult to distinguish between an attack of angina and a heart attack. Unlike a heart attack, angina is usually relieved by rest or by placing a tablet of glyceryl trinitrate (GTN) under the patient's tongue.

Signs and Symptoms of Heart Attack

1 Severe crushing chest pain, possibly radiating down one or both arms, or up into the jaw. The

pain will not be relieved by rest or the administration of GTN.

2 Facial pallor or 'ashen' appearance, sometimes with blueish colouring of the lips.

3 The skin may be cold and clammy to the touch and the casualty may be sweating profusely.

4 The patient may suffer from breathlessness, weakness and dizziness.

5 Nausea and vomiting may be present.

6 The pulse may be irregular and either slow or fast.

7 The patient may appear profoundly anxious.

8 The patient may collapse suddenly, possibly without warning.

Treatment of a heart attack

1 Keep the casualty as calm and as comfortable as possible. Loosen any tight clothing and place pillows behind his head and knees to support him in a half-sitting position.

2 Phone 999 for an ambulance (or ask somebody to do this for you so that you can remain with the casualty). Be prepared to resuscitate.

3 If ordinary aspirin is available, give the casualty one and ask him to chew and swallow it. Recent research has shown that aspirin given immediately after the onset of heart attack can improve the victim's chances of

recovery, perhaps by inhibiting further clotting in the coronary arteries.

Cardiac Arrest

Cardiac arrest is the term used to describe any sudden cessation of the heart, characterized by absence of pulse and breathing. Cardiac arrest may be the result of severe heart attack, anaphylactic shock, electric shock, poisoning (including drug overdose), hypothermia or suffocation.

During cardiac arrest, the brain and heart muscle are completely starved of oxygen, a state which can be tolerated only for a few minutes before permanent damage results. **Therefore it is vital that resuscitation procedures are instigated immediately**.

The ABC of Resuscitation

Resuscitation is the emergency action required when there is sustained interruption of the oxygen supply to the brain. In order that this vital oxygen supply may be restored, three vital conditions must be met:

A The **Airway** must be clear in order to permit oxygen-rich air to enter the lungs.

B There must be adequate **Breathing** taking place in order that the oxygen can enter the bloodstream.

C The blood must be pumped around the body providing effective **Circulation** to the brain and all body tissues.

When presented with an unconscious casualty, it is important to assess his condition **quickly** before attempting resuscitation. Therefore it is important to ask the following questions:

1 Is the patient unconscious with no evidence of pulse or breathing? If so: Dial 999 for an ambulance and carry out artificial ventilation and chest compression until the ambulance arrives.

2 Is the patient unconscious and not breathing but pulse is still present? If so: Give 10 breaths of artificial respiration and dial 999 for an ambulance. Continue artificial respiration until the ambulance arrives or spontaneous breathing is resumed. Check the pulse frequently.

3 Is the patient unconscious, but breathing, with pulse present? If so: Treat any obvious injuries, dial 999 for an ambulance and place the patient in the recovery position (see p.79).

Always proceed by following the ABC of Resuscitation.

A: Open the airway

1 Remove any visible obstructions from the mouth.

2 Placing two fingers under the casualty's chin, gently raise the jaw. Simultaneously, tilt the casualty's head well back by applying pressure to the forehead with your other hand.

Sometimes the airway may be blocked by the tongue as a result of loss of muscular control during unconsciousness, and this manoeuvre will lift the tongue clear.

B   Check for breathing

Place your face close to the casualty's mouth and listen and feel for breathing for a full 5 seconds. At the same time look along the chest and abdomen for signs of movement.

C   Check the circulation

If the heart is beating adequately, it will be possible to feel a **pulse** in the neck where the main carotid arteries pass on either side of the larynx on the way to the head. With the patient's head tilted back, slide your fingers between the Adam's Apple and the strap muscle and feel for the carotid pulse for five seconds.

If pulse and breathing are absent, you will need to commence artificial ventilation and chest compression immediately.

Mouth to Mouth or Artificial Ventilation

If the casualty is not breathing, but still has a pulse, then by breathing the exhaled air from your lungs into his you may be able to keep them adequately ventilated until help arrives.

1 Place the casualty flat on his back, and tilt the head back to open the airway unless you suspect Spinal Injury in which case lift the chin. Remove any obvious obstructions from the mouth. (Broken or loose dentures should be removed, but well-fitting dentures should remain in place).

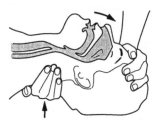

2 Pinch the nose between the index finger and thumb. Take a deep breath, then form a seal around the casualty's mouth with your own.

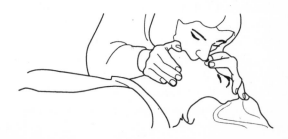

3 Blow steadily into the mouth until the chest rises. Each full inflation should take about two seconds.

4 Remove your lips from the casualty's and allow the chest to 'exhale' fully before giving a subsequent breath.

If the chest fails to rise:

1 Check that the head is tilted back correctly (see p.71).

2 Ensure that your lips are forming a proper seal around the patient's mouth.

3 Check that air is not escaping from the nostrils.

4 Check that the airway is not blocked by vomit or blood.

If an airway obstruction is suspected, then finger sweeps may be performed **on an adult**:

Grasp the tongue and lower jaw and pull gently upwards to open the mouth. Sweep the finger round the mouth and hook out any obstruction. (**This manoeuvre is not suitable for children**).

The first-aider should administer 10 breaths of artificial ventilation before phoning for an ambulance, then continue at a rate of approximately 10 breaths per minute until the casualty breathes spontaneously or medical help arrives.

Chest Compression

If the patient has no palpable carotid pulse and no breathing is present, then it is vital that you perform artificial ventilation and external chest compression to prevent brain damage which is likely to occur in just a few minutes. Artificial respiration and external chest compression are together known as **cardio-pulmonary resuscitation or CPR**.

1 Lie the patient flat on his back and feel for the point at which his lower ribs meet in the centre (the *xiphisternum*).

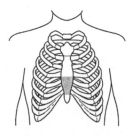

2 Place your left hand index and middle fingers over this point and the heel of your right hand on the breastbone or sternum above your fingers.

3 Place your left hand directly on top of your right hand interlocking the fingers. Pull the fingers away so that the heel of your right hand

is the only part in direct contact with the breastbone.

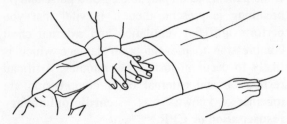

4 Keeping your arms straight, lean over the casualty and apply pressure to the breastbone. The intention is to depress and release the breastbone about 4–5cm or 1½–2 inches approximately 80 times per minute. Keep your hands in contact with the patient between compressions so that a smooth rhythm can be achieved. It may help to count aloud '1 and 2 and 3 and 4,' etc.

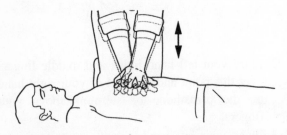

Compressing the chest in this way expels some of the blood from within the heart and forces it out into the tissues and around the body. As the pressure is released, more blood will be 'sucked' into the heart to replace that expelled.

The Sequence of CPR

The most effective sequence of CPR which can be performed by one person is 15 chest compressions followed by 2 breaths of artificial respiration. If two first-aiders are present the ratio should be 5 to 1.

Do not cease CPR unless:

1 The ambulance has arrived and paramedics take over.
2 The casualty moves or begins to groan, or his colour improves. If this occurs, then check immediately for a carotid pulse. If the pulse has returned, and the casualty is also breathing, place him in the recovery position (see p.79) until help arrives. If the pulse has restarted but breathing has not, then continue with artificial ventilation alone at a rate of 10 breaths per minute. Check the pulse at the end of every 10 ventilations, as you will need to restart full CPR again if it stops.
3 You are exhausted and cannot continue.

CPR for Children

Although it is rare for a child to suffer a cardiac arrest, it does occasionally happen and the first-aider should be aware that the main difference between treating a child and an adult is that the child will need to be given artificial ventilation for a full minute before dialling 999 for an ambulance. CPR can be performed on older children in much the same way as for adults, using a lighter and slightly faster technique, but must be modified as follows for use on children and babies.

1 **Airway:** Gently lift the chin and tilt the head to open the airway. **Do not perform finger sweeps or touch the back of the child's throat**. Any obvious food particles or other obstruction should be gently removed from the mouth.

2 **Breathing:** Look, feel and listen carefully for breathing. If it is absent, then begin artificial ventilation. This should be done as for adults, with the following exceptions.

a It is more effective to form a seal with your mouth round the child's mouth and nose than mouth alone.

b The rate of artificial ventilation will need to be

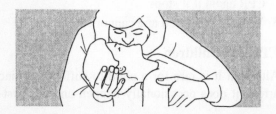

twice that for an adult—about 20 breaths per minute.

c Depending on the size of the child, you will need to vary the amount of air you breathe into the lungs to make the chest rise. A baby will only require tiny puffs, whereas an older child will need more.

3 **Circulation:** The carotid pulse is often hard to find in an infant—if so try the *brachial* pulse. You will find this half way between the shoulder and the elbow on the inner side of the arm. Press lightly with your index and middle fingers (perhaps using your thumb as a brace behind the arm) for a full 5 seconds. If no pulse is detected, you will need to begin chest compression. Use the adult technique if the child is large, but for babies and very young children it will need to be modified as follows:

a For a **baby**, imagine a line between his nipples and apply chest compression with two fingertips just below the line. Aim to depress the chest slightly less than 1 inch or two centimetres.

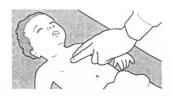

b For a **toddler** or small child, identify the correct position on the chest as per the adult technique, but use the heel of one hand only. Press to a depth of 3–4 cm or 1¹/₂ inches. In both cases, apply chest compressions at a rate of approximately 100 per minute, alternating 5 compressions with one breath.

Remember: If pulse and breathing are absent, artificial ventilation must be combined with chest compression. Call an ambulance as soon as possible.

The Recovery Position

An unconscious patient should always be placed in the recovery position, as the position of the head will prevent the tongue blocking the airway whilst allowing fluids to drain freely from the mouth. You should not leave an unconscious patient to call for help unless you have first placed him in the recovery position as follows:

1 Kneel beside the patient and open his airway by lifting the chin up and tilting the head. The arm nearest you should be placed at right angles to the body, with the elbow bent and the palm uppermost.

2 Bring the other arm across the patient's body and place his hand against his cheek. Hold the arm in this position.

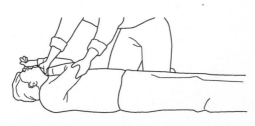

3 With your other hand, firmly grasp the far thigh and pull the knee up and towards you. Continue pulling until the patient is on his side with his hand still under his cheek.

4 Adjust the hand position and tilt the head back again if necessary to ensure that the airway remains open. The hand should keep the head in the correct position.

5 The upper leg should be bent so that the hip and the knee are both at right angles.

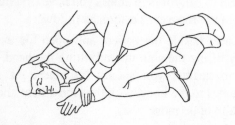

6 Call an ambulance immediately, and make frequent checks on the patient's pulse and breathing whilst you wait.

Poisoning

By poison we mean a substance which, if it enters the body can exert harmful effects, permanent or temporary. The routes by which a poison may enter the body are as follows:

1 **Swallowing**: May be accidental or deliberate (overdose) and includes a wide variety of substances from alcohol and illicit drugs to household cleaners or plants.

2 **Inhalation**: This can be of gases such as carbon monoxide, as well as solvents and vapours.

3 **Skin absorption**: Pesticides and insecticides may be absorbed in this way, and particularly strong chemicals may also cause burns.

4 **Injection into the skin**: This includes venom such as that injected by snakes and insects and also illicit drugs injected by abusers.

Detailed instruction on the treatment of specific types of poisoning is outwith the scope of this book, but in general the following steps should be taken:

1 Try to obtain an accurate history of the poisoning incident. If possible find out exactly

what the substance was, how much has been
ingested and how much time has elapsed since.

2 Obtain medical assistance immediately. **Never**
attempt to make the patient vomit as this may
cause further damage to the gastro-intestinal
tract and may even cause the patient to inhale
the vomit.

3 Place an unconscious patient in the recovery
position.

4 Send specimens of the toxin to the hospital
with the patient, if possible, as well as vomit
specimens. This will help in identification of
the toxin and the amount ingested.

Temperature Extremes

The body is designed to function at a temperature of between 36°C and 37.5°C (96.8°F and 99.5°F). Generally, the core temperature is kept constantly within these limits by a heat-regulating mechanism in the brain. Occasionally, the body temperature can rise or fall to a level whereby this mechanism can no longer effectively regulate the temperature resulting in the following conditions:

Hypothermia

Hypothermia occurs when the core temperature of the body falls to below 35° C (95°F). Once below 35°, shivering stops and the patient no longer feels cold but appears lethargic and apathetic. If the body temperature continues to drop, hypothermia sufferers may become increasingly confused and may even begin to experience sensations of heat and attempt to remove their clothing. At a temperature of below 30°C (86°F), the muscles become rigid and unconsciousness will eventually ensue. A body temperature of less than 27°C (80.6°F) will eventually cause cardiac arrest. Elderly people and babies are particularly

susceptible to hypothermia, but young, healthy
people can also be at risk if exposed to extremely
low temperatures for lengthy periods of time.

Treatment of Hypothermia

1 Bring the patient indoors and remove any wet
   clothing.
2 If indoors, and the casualty is capable of
   moving unaided, fill a bath with hot water
   (40°C/104°F) and completely immerse him in
   it. If the casualty is frail or elderly, allow him
   to warm up gradually in bed, well covered.
   Avoid using electric blankets and hot water
   bottles.
3 Give the patient something hot and sweet to
   drink. Avoid alcohol as it exacerbates
   hypothermia.
4 Call a doctor. If the casualty becomes
   unconscious, call an ambulance and be
   prepared to resuscitate.

Heat Exhaustion

Heat exhaustion usually occurs gradually and is
particularly common in those who have been
working or exercising vigorously in
unaccustomed heat. The symptoms are often
similar to those of shock (see p.96), due to the
excessive loss of fluids through perspiration. The

sufferer's temperature may be normal or only slightly raised, the skin cold and clammy and the pulse fast and weak. In addition, the loss of salt due to excessive perspiration may cause painful muscle cramps. The patient may also be hyperventilating.

Treatment of Heat Exhaustion

1 Remove the patient out of direct sunlight and heat to a shaded, cool place.
2 Ask the casualty to lie down and support her legs in a raised position.
3 Encourage her to drink plenty of weak salty water (about one teaspoon of salt per litre of water is sufficient).
4 If the patient recovers quickly, she should still be encouraged to see her doctor.
5 Should the patient become unconscious, place her in the recovery position (see p.79) and call an ambulance. While you are waiting for help to arrive, keep a check on the patient's pulse and breathing.

Heatstroke

Heatstroke often occurs rapidly resulting in unconsciousness within a few minutes, although there is sometimes a warning period when the patient may complain of feeling unwell or strange.

It occurs when the brain's 'thermostat' fails as a result of prolonged exposure to high temperature in the surroundings or illness with high fever.

Symptoms of Heatstroke

1 Dizziness, headache, discomfort and unease and confusion.
2 The skin will feel hot and dry and appear flushed.
3 The pulse will be fast and strong.
4 The patient may collapse and become unconscious.

Treatment of Heatstroke

1 Remove the casualty quickly to a cool place and remove his outer clothing. Summon medical help immediately.
2 If possible wrap the casualty in a sheet and keep it wet until his oral temperature falls to 38°C (100.4°F).
3 When the temperature has returned to a safe level, remove the wet sheet and substitute it for a dry one. Keep a close watch on the patient, and be prepared to repeat step 2 if the temperature rises again.
4. If the casualty becomes unconscious, place him in the recovery position (see p.79) and be prepared to resuscitate. Call an ambulance immediately.

Unconsciousness

Common Causes of Unconsciousness

1 Impairment of the blood supply to the brain. This may be a result of either
   a Fainting
   b Shock
   c Cardiac arrest
2 Impairment of oxygen supply to the brain. This may result from either
   a Choking
   b Suffocation
   c Carbon monoxide poisoning
3 Direct damage to the brain i.e. head injury.
4 Compression of the brain. This may be a result of either
   a Skull fracture
   b Infections
   c Tumour
   d Stroke
5 Alteration of the chemical balance of the brain's blood supply. This may be caused by either
   a Poisoning (including drugs and alcohol)

87

   b Low blood sugar (hypoglycaemia)

6 Other causes such as

   a Epilepsy

   b Abnormally high body temperature

   c Electrocution

First Aid for the Unconscious

Unconsciousness is caused by a variety of conditions which interrupt normal brain function. Unlike sleep, the casualty cannot be easily or completely roused in response to stimuli such as sound, or pain. The first-aider should always bear in mind that there is a danger that the airway will become blocked during unconsciousness either by vomit or by the tongue falling backwards causing an obstruction of the airway. Therefore always follow the following steps:

1 Lift the chin and gently tilt the head to open the airway. (If the patient begins to vomit, place in the recovery position.) If you suspect that there may be Spinal Injury open the airway by lifting the chin. Do not attempt to tilt the head.

2 Check the pulse and respiration. Be prepared to resuscitate if necessary.

3 Check the casualty for any heavy external bleeding or fractures and treat accordingly.

4 Place the patient in the recovery position

(see p.79) if you are satisfied that there is no
serious neck or spinal injury.

5 If full consciousness has not be regained
within 3 minutes, telephone 999 for an
ambulance.

DO NOT attempt to give the unconscious
patient anything by mouth.

DO NOT attempt to move the patient
unnecessarily, or to make him/her sit up.

Head Injuries and Loss of Consciousness

The brain is encased within the hard bony skull
and cushioned by cerebro-spinal fluid to protect it
from injury. It transmits impulses via the spinal
chord which runs down the neck and spine to all
the nerves of the body. The brain and spinal chord
are extremely fragile and incapable of repairing
themselves, hence the protection of the skull and
spine.

Fracture of the Skull

Although skull fracture is frequently indicative of
a   potentially   serious   and   life-threatening
condition, be aware that the real danger is damage
to the brain itself. There may be fragments of bony
skull causing pressure or compression on the brain
(depressed fracture) and the resulting indentation
of the skull may be missed as a result of swelling

in the scalp. Therefore all injuries to the head should be treated with the utmost caution and suspicion especially if any of the following signs of cerebral compression are present:

1 Vomiting, persistent headache or yawning.
2 Brief or partial loss of consciousness, or full unconsciousness.
3 Pupils of unequal sizes, which may enlarge and fail to constrict in response to light if compression increases.
4 One-sided paralysis or weakness of the face or body.
5 Irregular or noisy breathing, becoming increasingly slower.
6 Slow, strong pulse.
7 High temperature and flushed face.
8 Leakage of watery blood or straw-coloured fluid from the nose or ear.

Remember that an injury above chest level should be treated as a suspected Spinal Injury. In all cases, call 999 for an ambulance and treat as for unconsciousness whilst awaiting its arrival.

Diabetic Coma

Normally, an organ called the pancreas produces a hormone called insulin which regulates the level of sugar in our blood. In diabetes mellitus, the pancreas fails to perform this role adequately.

Sufferers may display symptoms such as tiredness, loss of weight, severe thirst, and passing large quantities of urine. Once diagnosed, patients can lead a relatively normal life with a few modifications. Mild diabetes may be controlled simply be restricting intake of carbohydrates in the diet, or by taking oral medication. More severe forms, however, will need to be controlled by regular injections of insulin and careful monitoring of energy intake.

Diabetic Emergencies—Hyper and Hypoglycaemia

If the blood sugar level falls below normal, then a condition known as hypoglycaemia is said to exist. Without adequate levels of sugar in the blood, the brain can no longer function normally. Most diabetics are aware of the steps they must take to prevent this occurring, and can usually identify the first symptoms of an attack and take the appropriate action—normally the ingestion of sugar or glucose tablets. However, if an attack becomes advanced, unconsciousness will eventually occur and failure to act quickly can result in brain damage.

How to Recognise a Hypoglycaemic Attack

1 The attack will usually be rapid in onset. The

patient may complain of weakness, tiredness, hunger or feeling faint. Ask if he is diabetic, or look for a medic-alert bracelet or warning card.

2 The patient may experience palpitations and muscle tremors.

3 If no sugar is taken, the patient may become confused or aggressive.

4 Skin will become cold, clammy and sweaty.

5 Breathing may become shallow.

6 Patient may eventually become unconscious.

Treatment of Hypoglycaemia

1 Aim to raise the blood sugar levels as quickly as possible by giving the victim sugary food or drink. Ascertain whether or not the patient carries a supply of Glucagon Injection for such emergencies, in which case follow the instructions enclosed. If there is no improvement within five minutes or...

2 If the victim is unconscious, place him in the recovery position and be prepared to resuscitate.

3 Call for an ambulance.

Hyperglycaemia

In hyperglycaemia, the pancreas fails to produce enough insulin to prevent excessive levels of

sugar in the blood. Once diagnosed, diabetics will
be able to prevent hyperglycaemia by balancing
their dietary intake of sugar and by regular insulin
injections.

Occasionally, hyperglycaemia can cause
unconsciousness, but the condition generally
develops gradually over a period of days or
weeks. The symptoms of hyperglycaemic coma
are as follows:

1 Dry skin
2 Faint smell of acetone (similar to nail varnish
   remover or mown grass) on the breath
3 Rapid pulse
4 Deep, laboured breathing.

Dial 999 for an ambulance or transport the
   patient to hospital immediately for treatment.

Shock and Allergic Reactions

An allergy is an abnormal response by the body to a specific stimulus or allergen. These can be familiar, everyday substances such as house dust, pollen or animal fur causing mild symptoms such as sneezing, itchiness or a rash. Hay fever, for instance is an allergic response to pollens in the air and is most commonly experienced in the summer months. Similarly, many people may suffer unpleasant allergic reactions after ingesting particular foods. Shellfish, nuts and eggs are often the culprits, and most sufferers quickly manage to identify those foods which cause the reaction and thereafter avoid them. Sometimes, patients can also experience an allergic response to some drugs such as penicillin, and medical practitioners will always bear this in mind when prescribing medication.

Although allergies can be extremely unpleasant and distressing for the sufferer, they will rarely necessitate first aid or emergency treatment. However, a patient may occasionally experience a severe and life-threatening reaction to an allergen. This is known as anaphylactic shock and requires urgent medical attention. This reaction can occur in response to bee or wasp stings or the ingestion of nuts or any food which causes allergy in the sufferer and can therefore be extremely difficult to diagnose.

Anaphylactic Shock

1 Does the patient's skin have a rash or red blotches (hives)?

2 Is there any swelling on any part of the patient's body, but particularly on the face, the lips or the tongue?

3 Is he having difficulty in breathing? This may indicate swelling in the airway.

4 Is he experiencing tightness in his chest?

5 Is his skin colour normal or does it appear greyish or even blue?

6 Is the patient unconscious or suffering from seizures?

7 Can his pulse be felt? Is it weak or rapid?

Any of the above symptoms can develop within a few moments of the initial exposure to the allergen. The treatment for severe anaphylactic shock is the administration of the drug adrenaline and oxygen. Increasingly, allergy suffer-ers identified as being at risk of anaphylactic shock will be issued with pre-packed injections of adrenaline which are quick and simple to use, so it is sensible to check whether or not your patient is thus equipped. Otherwise, there is no specific treatment other than remaining with your patient until medical help arrives. He should be kept in a comfortable upright position to assist breathing, unless he loses consciousness, in which case the recovery position is preferred.

Shock

When referred to in medical emergency, shock is taken to signify a life-threatening condition caused by the failure of the circulatory system to pump blood around the body. Internal and external bleeding can cause this, as can heart attack, anaphylactic shock and excessive loss of body fluids such as that which occurs in diarrhoea or severe burns. The body tries to maximise the use of remaining body fluids by withdrawing them from the surface and extremities of the body to the centre. This can progressively produce the following symptoms:

1 The patient's skin becomes cold, grey and clammy as the body attempts to divert blood supplies to the vital organs.
2 The pulse becomes rapid as the heart works harder to circulate the reduced volume of blood.

3 The pulse becomes weaker and may become irregular as the blood volume and pressure fall.

4 The patient becomes weak and giddy as oxygen fails to reach the muscles and brain.

5 The patient's breathing becomes rapid and shallow, and he may appear to be attempting to yawn or gulp in air ('air hunger').

6 The patient may complain of nausea and actually vomit.

7 The patient may experience thirst as the brain senses that the body needs to make up a shortfall in fluid.

8 The patient may become restless and agitated as the oxygen supply to the brain deteriorates.

9 The patient will lose consciousness, and the pulse at the wrist may become unpalpable.

10 The heart will stop.

It is vital to identify and treat the causes of shock immediately.

Always summon medical help at the earliest possible opportunity, but it may be possible to slow the progression of shock by taking prompt action to stop bleeding from an open wound.

MEDICAL TERMS

A

ABDOMEN the region of the body which lies below the THORAX, being divided from it by the DIAPHRAGM, and above the pelvis. The abdominal cavity contains the DIGESTIVE ORGANS (e.g. the STOMACH and INTESTINES), the EXCRETORY ORGANS (BLADDER and KIDNEYS) and, in females, the REPRODUCTIVE ORGANS (WOMB and OVARIES).

ABORTION the removal of an embryo or foetus from the womb, either by natural expulsion or by human intervention, before it is considered to be viable at the 24th week of pregnancy. An abortion may be *spontaneous*, and this is commonest during the first three months of pregnancy and is thought to be most often associated with abnormalities in the foetus. Or, an abortion may be *induced*, when it is also known as *therapeutic*, or *termination of pregnancy*, and is carried out for medical or social reasons.

ABSCESS a collection of pus at a localized site anywhere in the body resulting from an infection caused by bacteria. Treatment is by the surgical opening of the abscess and by the administration of ANTIBIOTICS.

ACQUIRED a condition or malady that is not CONGENITAL but arises after birth.

ACUTE a disease or condition which is short-lived, and which starts rapidly with severe symptoms.

ADENITIS refers to inflammation of one or more glands.

ADENOIDS a clump of lymphoid tissue situated at the back of the nose (in the nasopharynx). The adenoids may become swollen as a result of persistent throat infections, and obstruct breathing through the nose.

ADRENAL GLANDS each of the two kidneys within the body bears an adrenal gland upon its upper surface. The adrenal glands, also known as suprarenal glands, are important ENDOCRINE organs, producing HORMONES that regulate various body functions. Each adrenal gland has two parts, an outer cortex and an inner medulla which secrete a variety of hormones. Two of the most important ones are ADRENALINE and CORTISONE.

ADRENALINE a very important hormone produced by the medulla of the adrenal glands which, when released, prepares the body for 'fright, flight or fight' by increasing the depth and rate of respiration, raising the heartbeat rate and improving muscle performance. It also has an inhibitive effect on the processes of digestion and excretion. It can be used medically in a variety of ways, for instance in the treatment of bronchial asthma where it relaxes the airways, and also to stimulate the heart when there is cardiac arrest. Adrenaline is also known as epinephrine.

ADULT RESPIRATORY DISTRESS SYNDROME describes the condition of severe respiratory failure brought about by a number of different disorders. There is a lack of oxygen in the blood, which exhibits itself by imparting a blue tinge to the skin, and rapid breathing and pulse rate. The syndrome may be caused by physical damage to the lungs, by infection or by an adverse reaction following surgery or transfusion. It is often fatal.

AIDS this refers to Acquired *Immune Deficiency Syndrome*. The causal agent is the human immunodeficiency virus known as HIV. The virus has been found in blood, other body fluids, semen and cervical secretions and is mainly transmitted by sexual activity. The HIV virus affects the T-lymphocytes of the immune system, and leaves the patient increasingly unable to resist certain infections and tumours which are particularly associated with AIDS. Although they may take a long time to develop, these infections eventually prove to be fatal and at the present time there is no known cure for AIDS.

AIR EMBOLISM a bubble of air in a blood vessel which interferes with the outward flow of blood from the right ventricle of the heart. The air may enter the circulation after an injury, surgery or infusion into a vein. The symptoms are chest pain and breathlessness leading to acute heart failure.

AIR PASSAGES these are all the openings and passages through which air enters and is taken into the lungs. These are the nose, pharynx (throat), larynx, trachea (windpipe) and bronchial tubes. Air entering via this route has dust particles removed, and is warmed and moistened before entering the lungs.

ALIMENTARY CANAL the whole of the passage along which food is passed starting at the mouth and ending at the anus.

ALLERGEN any substance, usually a protein, which causes a hypersensitive (allergic) reaction in a person who is exposed to the allergen. There are a great variety of allergens which cause reactions in different tissues and body functions. The respiratory system and skin are often affected.

ALLERGY a state of hypersensitivity in an affected individual to a particular allergen, which produces a characteristic response whenever the person is exposed to the substance. In an unaffected person, antibodies present in the bloodstream destroy their particular antigens (ALLERGENS). However, in an affected individual this reaction causes some cell damage and there is a release of

substances such as histamine and bradykin which cause the allergic reaction. Examples of allergies are dermatitis, hay fever, asthma and the severe response known as ANAPHYLAXIS.

ALVEOLUS (*plural* **ALVEOLI**) a small sac or cavity which in numbers forms the alveolar sacs at the end of the BRONCHIOLES in the lungs. Each alveolus is fed by a rich blood supply via capillaries (*see* CAPILLARY) and is lined with a moist membrane where oxygen and carbon dioxide, the respiratory gases, are exchanged. The alveolar sacs provide an enormous surface area for efficient respiration.

AMNESIA loss of memory which may be partial or total. *Anterograde* amnesia is the loss of memory of recent events following a trauma of some kind. *Retrograde* amnesia is the inability to remember events that preceded a trauma. Other types of amnesia are *post-traumatic* and *hysterical* and more than one kind may be experienced by an individual.

ANAEMIA a decrease in the ability of the blood to carry oxygen due to a reduction in the number of red blood cells or in the amount of haemoglobin which they contain. Haemoglobin is the pigment within the red blood cells which binds to oxygen. There are a number of different types of anaemia and a variety of reasons for it, and treatment depends upon the underlying cause.

ANAESTHESIA a loss of sensation or feeling in the whole or part of the body, usually relating to the administration of anaesthetic drugs so that surgery can be performed.

ANALGESIA a state of reduced reaction to pain, but without loss of consciousness. It may be due to drugs(analgesics) or it may happen accidentally should nerves become diseased or damaged.

ANAPHYLAXIS a response exhibited by a hypersensitive individual when confronted with a particular ANTIGEN. It results from the release of histamine in body tissues following the antigen-antibody reaction within cells. An allergic reaction is an example of mild anaphylaxis. Anaphylatic shock is a much rarer and more serious condition which can follow the injection of drugs or vaccines, or a bee sting, to which the individual is hypersensitive. Its onset is immediate and results from a widespread release of histamine in the body. The symptoms include severe breathing difficulties, swelling (OEDEMA), a fall in blood pressure, acute URTICARIA and heart failure. Death may follow if the individual is not soon treated with adrenaline by injection.

ANEURYSM a balloon-like swelling of the wall of an artery which occurs when it becomes weakened or damaged in some way. There may be a congenital weakness in the muscular wall of the artery involved, as is often the case within the brain. Damage may also be the result of infection, particularly SYPHILIS, or degenerative conditions e.g. ATHEROMA.

ANGINA a suffocating, choking pain, usually used in reference to angina pectoris, which is felt in the chest. The pain is felt or brought on by exercise and relieved by rest, and occurs when the blood supply to the heart muscle is inadequate. During exercise the demand for blood (supplied by the coronary arteries) is increased and if the supply is insufficient, because the arteries are damaged, chest pain results. The coronary arteries may be damaged by ATHEROMA, the most common cause. Angina pectoris is usually first treated with drugs but if the condition worsens, coronary-artery

by-pass surgery may need to be performed.

ANGIOMA a clump of distended blood vessels pushing onto the surface of the brain. It may cause epilepsy and occasionally a vessel may burst to cause a SUBARACHNOID HAEMORRHAGE.

ANOXIA the condition when the body tissues do not receive sufficient oxygen. It may be due to high altitudes (and thus lower atmospheric pressure), a lack of red blood cells, or a disease such as PNEUMONIA which limits the amount of oxygen reaching the lung surfaces and therefore reduces that available for transfer to the blood.

ANTIBIOTIC a substance, derived from a micro-organism which kills or inhibits the multiplication of other micro-organisms, usually bacteria or fungi. Well-known examples are penicillin and streptomycin.

ANTIBODIES protein substances of the GLOBULIN type which are produced by the lymphoid tissue and circulate in the blood. They react with their corresponding ANTIGENS and neutralize them, rendering them harmless. Antibodies are produced against a wide variety of antigens and these reactions are responsible for IMMUNITY and ALLERGY.

ANTICONVULSANTS drugs which are used to reduce the severity of epileptic fits (convulsions) or to prevent them from occurring.

ANTIDOTE a substance which counter-acts the effect of a particular poison.

ANTIGENS any substances which cause the formation by the body of ANTIBODIES to neutralize their effect. Antigens are often protein substances, regarded as 'foreign' and 'invading' by the body, and elicit the production of antibodies against them. *See* ALLERGEN, ALLERGY and ANAPHYLAXIS.

ANTIHISTAMINES drugs which

counteract the effects of histamine release in the body. They are widely used to treat allergic reactions of various sorts, particularly to relieve skin conditions. Those taken by mouth have a sedative effect and so care must be taken while they are being used.

ANTISEPTICS substances which prevent the growth of disease-causing micro-organisms such as bacteria, and are applied to the skin to prevent infection and to cleanse wounds. Examples are iodine and crystal violet.

ANTISERUM a serum that is usually prepared from horses, which contains a high concentration of antibody against a particular antigen. It is injected to give immunity against a particular disease or toxin.

ANUS the opening of the alimentary canal at the opposite end from the mouth, through which faeces are voided. The anus is at the lower end of the bowel and its opening is controlled by two muscles, the internal and external sphincters.

AORTA the major large artery of the body which arises from the left ventricle of the heart and which carries blood to all areas. The other arteries of the body are all derived from the aorta.

APHASIA speechlessness caused by disease or injury to those parts of the brain which govern the activities involved in speech-making. It is caused by THROMBOSIS, EMBOLISM or HAEMORRHAGE of a blood vessel within the brain as in a STROKE, or by a TUMOUR. It may be temporary if the blood supply is not permanently damaged, but often the power of speech continues to be impaired and is associated with other intellectual disorders.

APHONIA the loss of the voice which may be caused by disease or by damage to the LARYNX or mouth or to nerves controlling throat

muscles, or may result from hysteria.

APNOEA a temporary halt in breathing which may result from a number of different causes. Apnoea is quite common in newborn infants and can be registered by an apnoea monitor which sounds an alarm if the baby ceases to breathe.

APPENDICITIS inflammation of the vermiform APPENDIX which, in its acute form, is the most common abdominal emergency in the western world, usually requiring treatment by appendicectomy. It is most common in young people during their first 20 years, and the symptoms include abdominal pain which may move about, appetite loss, sickness and diarrhoea. If not treated the appendix can become the site of an ABSCESS, or gangrenous, which eventually may result in PERITONITIS. This arises because infected material spreads from the burst appendix into the peritoneal cavity.

APPENDIX a blind-ended tube which is an appendage of various organs within the body. It normally refers to the vermiform appendix which is about 9 to 10 cm long and projects from the CAECUM (a pouch) of the large intestine. It has no known function and can become the site of infection probably as the result of obstruction. *See* APPENDICITIS.

ARRYTHMIA any disturbance in the normal rhythm of heartbeat. The built-in pacemaker of the heart is the sinoatrial node situated in the wall of the right atrium, which itself is regulated by the AUTONOMIC NERVOUS SYSTEM. The electrical impulses produced by the pacemaker control the rate and rhythm of heartbeat. Arrythmias occur when these electrical impulses are disturbed.

ARTERIOLE a small branch of an artery leading to a capillary.

ARTERITIS inflammation of an artery.

ARTERY a blood vessel which

carries blood away from the heart. Oxygenated (bright red) blood is carried by the arteries to all parts of the body. However, the pulmonary arteries carry dark, unoxygenated blood from the heart to the lungs. An artery has thick, elastic walls which are able to expand and contract, and contain smooth muscle fibres. This smooth muscle is uder the control of the SYMPATHETIC NERVOUS SYSTEM.

ARTHRITIS inflammation of the joints or spine, the symptoms of which are pain and swelling, restriction of movement, redness and warmth of the skin. There are many different causes of arthritis including OSTEOARTHRITIS, RHEUMATOID ARTHRITIS, TUBERCULOSIS and RHEUMATIC FEVER.

ARTIFICIAL RESPIRATION an emergency procedure carried out when normal respiration has ceased in order to artificially ventilate the lungs, usually referred to as 'mouth-to-mouth resus-citation.' In hospital where a seriously ill person is unable to breathe unaided, artificial respiration is achieved by means of a machine known as a ventilator.

ASTHMA a condition characterized by breathing difficulties caused by narrowing of the airways (bronchi, see BRONCHUS) of the lung. Asthma may occur at any age but usually begins in early childhood, and is a hypersensitive response which can be brought on by exposure to a variety of ALLERGENS, exercise, stress or infections. An asthma sufferer may have other hypersensitive conditions such as eczema and hay fever, and it may be prevalent within a family. Treatment involves the use of drugs to dilate the airways (bronchodilators) and also inhaled corticosteroids.

ATAXIA a loss of co-ordination in the limbs due to a disorder of the CENTRAL NERVOUS SYSTEM. There may be a disease of the sensory nerves

(sensory ataxia) or of the CEREBELLUM (cerebellar ataxia). An ataxic person produces clumsy movements and lacks fine control.

ATHEROMA a degenerative condition of the arteries. The inner and middle coats of the arterial walls become scarred and fatty deposits (CHOLESTEROL) are built up at these sites. The blood circulation is impaired and it may lead to such problems as ANGINA pectoris, stroke and heart attack. The condition is associated with the western lifestyle. i.e. lack of exercise, smoking, obesity and too high an intake of animal fats.

ATHEROSCLEROSIS similar to ATHEROMA being a degenerative disease of the arteries associated with fatty deposits on the inner walls leading to reduced blood flow.

ATHLETE'S FOOT a fungal infection of the skin particularly occurring between the toes and often due to ringworm.

ATRIUM (*pl.* **ATRIA**) one of the two thin-walled, upper chambers of the heart, which receive blood from major veins. The right atrium receives (deoxygenated) blood from the venae cavae and the left atrium is supplied with (oxygenated) blood from the pulmonary vein. (Atria also refers to various other chambers in the body.)

AURAL anything relating to the ear.

AURICLE the external part of the ear of flap known as the pinna. Also, an ear-shaped appendage of the ATRIUM of the heart.

AUTOANTIBODY an antibody produced by the body against one of its own tissues which is a feature of AUTOIMMUNE DISEASE.

AUTOIMMUNE DISEASE one of a number of conditions resulting from the production of antibodies by the body which attack its own tissues. For reasons which are not understood the immune system loses the ability to distinguish between 'self' and 'non-self'. Autoimmune disease is currently thought to be the cause of a number of disorders including acquired haemolytic anaemia.

AUTOIMMUNITY a failure of the immune system in which the body develops antibodies that attack components or substances belonging to itself. *See* AUTOANTIBODY, AUTOIMMUNE DISEASE.

AUTONOMIC NERVOUS SYSTEM the part of the nervous system which controls body functions that are not under conscious control, e.g. the heartbeat and other smooth muscles and glands. It is divided into the SYMPATHETIC and PARASYMPATHETIC NERVOUS SYSTEMS.

B

BACILLUS (*plural* bacilli) a term for any bacterium that is rod-shaped. Also a genus of gram-positive (*see* GRAM'S STAIN) bacteria that includes *B. anthracis*, the cause of anthrax.

BACKBONE *see* SPINAL COLUMN.

BACTERIA (*singular* bacterium) single-celled organisms that underpin all life sustaining processes. GRAM'S STAIN is a test used to distinguish between the two types (Gram positive and Gram negative). They are also identified by shape: spiral, (spirilli), rod-like (bacilli), spherical (cocci), comma-shaped (vibrid) and the spirochaetal that are corkscrew-like. Bacteria are the key agents in the chemical cycles of carbon, oxygen, nitrogen and sulphur.

BACTERICIDE something that kills bacteria, but used especially when referring to drugs and antiseptics.

BACTERIOPHAGE a virus that attacks a BACTERIUM. The phage replicates in the host which is ultimately destroyed as new phages are released. Each phage is specific to a certain bacterium and uses are found in genetic engineering in cloning and certain manufacturing processes.

BASAL GANGLION GREY MATTER at the base of the CEREBRUM that is involved in the subconscious control of voluntary movement.

BENIGN used most frequently with reference to tumours, meaning not harmful.

BILE a viscous, bitter fluid produced by the LIVER and stored in the GALL BLADDER. It is an alkaline solution of bile salts, pigments, some mineral salts and CHOLESTEROL which aids in fat digestion and absorption of nutrients. Discharge of bile into the intestine is increased after food and of the amount secreted each day (up to one litre), most is reabsorbed with the food, passing back into the blood to circulate back to the liver. If the flow of bile into the intestine is restricted, it stays in the blood, resulting in jaundice.

BILE DUCT a duct that carries BILE from the liver. The main duct is the hepatic which joins the cystic duct from the GALL BLADDER to form the common bile duct which drains into the small INTESTINE.

BIOPSY an adjunct to diagnosis which involves removing a small sample of living tissue from the body for examination under the microscope. The technique is particularly important in differentiating between benign and malignant tumours. A biopsy can be undertaken with a hollow needle inserted into the relevant organ.

BLADDER a sac of fibrous and muscular tissue that contains secretions and which can increase and decrease in capacity. Discharge of the contents is through a narrow opening (*see for example* GALL BLADDER *and* URINARY ORGANS).

BLINDNESS being unable to see, a

condition which may vary from a
total lack of light perception (total
blindness) through degrees of visual
impairment. The commonest causes
of blindness are GLAUCOMA, senile
CATARACT, vitamin A deficiency
(night blindness) and DIABETES
MELLITUS.

BLOOD a suspension of red blood
cells (or corpuscles) called
erythrocytes, white blood cells
(leucocytes) and platelets (small
disc-shaped cells involved in BLOOD
CLOTTING) in a liquid medium, blood
PLASMA. The circulation of blood
through the body provides a
mechanism for transporting
substances. Its functions include:
1) carrying oxygenated blood from
the heart to all tissues via the arteries
while the veins return deoxygenated
blood to the heart.
2) carrying essential nutrients, e.g.
glucose, fats and amino acids to all
parts of the body.
3) removing the waste products of
metabolism - ammonia and carbon
dioxide, to the liver where urea is
formed and then transported by the
blood to the kidneys for excretion.
4) carrying important molecules, e.g.
hormones, to their target cells.
The red blood cells, produced in the
bone marrow, are haemoglobin-
containing discs while the white
varieties vary in shape and are
produced in the marrow and
lymphoid tissue. The plasma
comprises water, proteins and
electrolytes and forms approximately
half the blood volume.

BLOOD CLOT a hard mass of
blood platelets, trapped red blood
cells and fibrin. After tissue damage,
blood vessels in the area are
constricted and a plug forms to seal
the damaged are. The plug formation
is initiated by an ENZYME released by
the damaged blood vessels and
platelets.

BLOOD GROUPS the division and

classification of people into one of
four main groups based upon the
presence of ANTIGENS on the surface
of the red blood cells (corpuscles).
The classifying reaction depends
upon the SERUM of one person's
blood agglutinating (clumping
together) the red blood cells of
someone else. The antigens, known
as agglutinogens react with
antibodies (agglutinins) in the serum.
There are two agglutinogens termed A
and B and two agglutinins called anti-
A and anti-B. This gives rise to four
groups: corpuscles with no
agglutinogens, group O; with A;
with B and with both A and B (hence
blood group AB). The agglutinin
groups match those of the
agglutinogens, thus a person of
blood group B has anti-A serum in
their blood. It is vital that blood
groups are matched for transfusion
because incompatibility will produce
blood clotting.
The Rhesus factor is another antigen
(named after the Rhesus monkey
which has a similar antigen), those
with it being Rh-positive and those
without Rh-negative. About 85% of
people are Rh-positive. If a Rh-
negative person receives Rh-positive
blood, or if a Rh-positive foetus is
exposed to antibodies to the factor in
the blood of the Rh-negative mother,
then HAEMOLYSIS occurs in the foetus
and newborn child. This may cause
the stillbirth of the child, or jaundice
after birth. Testing of pregnant
women is thus essential.

BLOOD POISONING *see*
SEPTICAEMIA.

BLOOD PRESSURE the pressure
of the blood on the heart and blood
vessels in the system of circulation.
Also the pressure that has to be
applied to an artery to stop the pulse
beyond the pressure point.
Blood pressure peaks at a heart beat
(SYSTOLE) and falls in between
(DIASTOLE). The systolic pressure in

young adults is equivalent to approximately 120mm mercury (and 70mm in diastole). The pressure also depends upon the hardness and thickness of vessel walls and blood pressure tends to increase with age as arteries thicken and harden.

A temporary rise in blood pressure may be precipitated by exposure to cold; a permanent rise by kidney disease and other disorders. A lower blood pressure can be induced by a hot bath or caused by exhaustion. The instrument used to measure blood pressure is the SPHYGMOMA-NOMETER.

BLOOD SUGAR glucose concentration in the blood for which the typical value is 3.5 to 5.5 mmol/l (millimoles per litre). *See also* HYPOGLYCAEMIA and HYPERGLYCAEMIA.

BLOOD TRANSFUSION the replacement of blood lost due to injury, surgery, etc. A patient may receive whole blood or a component e.g. packed red cells (red blood cells separated from the PLASMA, used to counteract anaemia and restore HAEMOGLOBIN levels). Blood from donors is matched to the recipient for BLOOD GROUP and haemoglobin. Donor blood can be stored for three weeks before use if kept just a few degrees above freezing after which the platelets, leucocytes and some red blood cells become non-viable. Plasma and serum are also transfused and in the dried form, plasma can be stored for up to five years.

BLOOD VESSEL the veins and arteries and their smaller branchings, venules and arterioles, through which blood carried to and from the heart.

BOIL (or furuncle) a skin infection in a hair follicle or gland that produces inflammation and pus. The infection is often due to the bacterium *Staphylococcus*, but healing is generally quick upon release of the pus or administration of antibiotics. Frequent occurrence of boils is usually investigated to ensure the patient is not suffering from DIABETES MELLITUS.

BONE the hard connective tissue that with CARTILAGE forms the skeleton. Bone has a matrix of COLLAGEN fibres with bone salts (crystalline calcium phosphate or hydroxyapatite, in which are the bone cells, OSTEOBLASTS and OSTEOCYTES). The bone cells form the matrix.

There are two types of bone: compact or dense, forming the shafts of long bones and spongy or cancellous which occurs on the inside and at the ends of long bones, and also forms the short bones. Compact bone is a hard tube covered by the periosteum (a membrane) and enclosing the marrow and contains very fine canals (*see* HAVERSIAN CANALS) around which the bone is structured in circular plates (*see also* BONE DISEASES, BONE MARROW).

BONE MARROW a soft tissue found in the spaces of bones. In young animals all bone marrow, the red marrow, produces blood cells. In older animals the marrow in long bones is replaced by yellow marrow which contains a large amount of fat and does not produce blood cells. In mature animals the red marrow occurs in the ribs, sternum, vertebrae and the ends of the long bones (e.g. the femur). The red marrow contains MYELOID tissue with ERYTHROBLASTS from which red blood cells develop. LEUCOCYTES also form from the myeloid tissue and themselves give rise to other cell types.

BRACHIAL adjective meaning 'of the upper arm', hence brachial artery etc.

BRADYCARDIA slowness of the heart-beat and pulse to below 60 per minute.

BRAIN the part of the CENTRAL

NERVOUS SYSTEM contained within the cranium and is connected via the spinal cord to the remainder of the nervous system. The brain interprets information received from sense organs and emits signals to control muscles. The brain comprises distinct areas: the CEREBRUM, CEREBELLUM, PONS, MEDULLA OBLONGATA and mid-brain or mesencephalon. GREY MATTER and WHITE MATTER make up the brain, in different arrangements, and a dense network of blood vessels supplies the grey matter and both blood vessels and nerve cells are supported by a fibrous network, the NEUROGLIA. Three membranes (the MENINGES) separate the brain from the skull and between each pair is a fluid-filled space to cushion the brain. There are twelve nerves connected to the brain mainly in the region of the brain stem and four arteries carrying blood to the brain. Two veins drain the central portion and many small veins open into venous SINUSES which connect with the internal jugular vein.

BRAINSTEM DEATH (or BRAIN DEATH) a complete and continuous absence of the vital reflexes controlled by centres in the brainstem (breathing, pupillary responses, etc.). Tests are performed by independent doctors, repeated after an interval, before death is formally confirmed.

BREAST the MAMMARY GLAND that produces milk. Each breast has a number of compartments with lobules surrounded by fatty tissue and muscle fibres. Milk formed in the lobules gathers in branching tubes or ducts that together form lactiferous ducts. Near the nipple the ducts form ampullae (small 'reservoirs') from which the ducts discharge through the nipple.

BREATHLESSNESS is caused fundamentally by any condition that depletes blood oxygen resulting in excessive and/or laboured breathing to gain more air. The causes are numerous, ranging from lung diseases or conditions (PNEUMONIA, EMPHYSEMA, BRONCHITIS) to heart conditions and obesity. In children, narrowing of the air passages is a cause, as is ASTHMA.

BRITTLE BONE DISEASE see OSTEOGENESIS IMPERFECTA.

BRONCHIOLE very fine tubes occurring as branches of the bronchi (see BRONCHUS). The bronchioles end in alveoli (see ALVEOLUS) where carbon dioxide and oxygen are exchanged.

BRONCHITIS occurring in two forms, acute and chronic, bronchitis is the inflammation of the bronchi. Bacteria or viruses cause the acute form which is typified by the symptoms of the common cold initially, but develops with painful coughing, wheezing, throat and chest pains and the production of purulent (pus-containing) mucus. If the infection spreads to the BRONCHIOLES (bronchiolitis) the consequences are more serious as the body is deprived of oxygen. Antibiotics and expectorants can relieve the symptoms.
Chronic bronchitis is identified by an excessive production of mucus and may be due to recurrence of the acute form. It is a common cause of death among the elderly and there are several parameters of direct consequence to its cause: excessive smoking of cigarettes; cold, damp climate; obesity; respiratory infections. Damage to the bronchi and other complications may occur giving rise to constant breathlessness.

BRONCHODILATOR drugs used to relax the SMOOTH MUSCLE of the bronchioles, thus increasing their diameter and the air supply to the lungs. They are used in the treatment of ASTHMA.

BRONCHUS air passages supported by rings of cartilage. Two bronchi

branch off from the TRACHEA and
these split into further bronchi. The
two main bronchi branch to form
five lobar bronchi, then twenty
segmental bronchi and so on.

BUCCAL generally pertaining to the
mouth, specifically the inside of the
cheek or the gum next to the cheek.

BURNS burns and scalds show
similar symptoms and require
similar treatment, the former being
caused by dry heat, the latter moist
heat. Burns may also be due to
electric currents and chemicals.
Burns are categorized by as either
superficial, where sufficient tissue
remains to ensure skin regrows, or
deep where GRAFTING will be
necessary.
Severe injuries can prove dangerous
because of shock due to fluid loss at
the burn. For minor burns and
scalds, treatment involves holding
the affected area under cold water. In
more severe cases antiseptic
dressings are normally applied and in
very severe cases hospitalization is
required.

C

CAECUM an expanded, blind-
ended sac at the start of the large
intestine between the small intestine
and colon. the small intestine and
vermiform appendix open into the
caecum.

CAESARIAN SECTION a surgical
operation to deliver a baby by means
of an incision through the abdomen
and uterus. It is performed when
there is a risk to the health of the
baby or mother through normal
delivery, both as a planned and as an
emergency procedure.

CALLUS material which forms
around the end of a broken bone
containing bone-forming cells,
cartilage and connective tissue.

Eventually this tissue becomes
calcified.

CANCER a widely-used term
describing any form of malignant
tumour. Characteristically, there is
an uncontrolled and abnormal
growth of cancer cells which invade
surrounding tissues and destroy
them. Cancer cells may spread
throughout the body via the blood
stream or lymphatic system, a
process known as METASTASIS, and set
up secondary growths elsewhere.
There are known to be a number of
different causes of cancer including
cigarette smoking, radiation,
ultraviolet light, some viruses and
possibly the presence of cancer
GENES (oncogenes). Treatment
depends upon the site of the cancer
but involves radiotherapy,
chemotherapy and surgery, and
survival rates in affected people are
showing encouraging improvements.

CAPILLARY a fine blood vessel
which communicates with an
ARTERIOLE or VENULE. Capillaries form
networks in most tissues and have
walls which are only one cell thick.
There is a constant exchange of
substances (oxygen, carbon dioxide,
nutrients, etc.) between the
capillaries, arterioles and venules
supplying the needs of the
surrounding tissues.

CAPSULE a sheath of connective
tissue or membrane surrounding an
organ. The adrenal gland, kidney and
spleen are all housed within a
capsule. A JOINT capsule is a fibrous
tissue sheath surrounding various
joints. A capsule is also used to
describe a small, gelatinous pouch
containing a drug, which can be
swallowed.

CARBON DIOXIDE also known as
carbonic acid, this is a gas formed in
the tissues as a result of metabolic
processes within the body. Medically,
carbon dioxide is used combined with
oxygen during anaesthesia.

CARBON MONOXIDE (CO) an odourless and colourless gas which is highly dangerous when inhaled, leading to carbon monoxide poisoning. In the blood it has a very great affinity for oxygen and converts haemoglobin into carboxyhaemoglobin. The tissues of the body are quickly deprived of oxygen because there is no free haemoglobin left to pick it up in the lungs. Carbon monoxide is present in coal gas fumes and vehicle exhaust emissions. The symptoms of poisoning include giddiness, flushing of the skin (due to carboxyhaemoglobin in the blood which is bright red), nausea, headache, raised respiratory and pulse rate and eventual coma, respiratory failure and death. An affected person must be taken into the fresh air and given oxygen and artificial respiration if required.

CARCINOGEN any substance which causes damage to tissue cells likely to result in cancer. Various substances are known to be *carcinogenic* including tobacco smoke, asbestos and ionizing radiation.

CARCINOMA a cancer of the EPITHELIUM, i.e. the tissue that lines the body's internal organs and skin.

CARDIAC ARREST the failure and stopping of the pumping action of the heart. There is a loss of consciousness and breathing and the pulse ceases. Death follows very rapidly unless the heart beat can be restored, and methods of achieving this include external CARDIAC MASSAGE, artificial respiration, DEFIBRILLATION and direct cardiac massage.

CARDIAC CYCLE the whole sequence of events which produces a heart beat which normally takes place in less than one second. The atria (*see* ATRIUM) contract together and force the blood into the ventricles (DIASTOLE). These then also contract (SYSTOLE) and blood exits the heart and is pumped around the body. As the ventricles are contracting the atria relax and fill up with blood once again.

CARDIAC MASSAGE a means of restoring the heart beat if this activity has suddenly ceased. Direct cardiac massage, which is only feasible if the person is in hospital, involves massaging the heart by hand through an incision in the chest wall. Another method, used in conjunction with artificial respiration, is by rhythmic compression of the chest wall while the person is laid on his or her back.

CARDIAC MUSCLE specialized muscle unique to the heart, consisting of branching, elongated fibres possessing the ability to contract and relax continuously.

CARDIOMYOPATHY any disease or disorder of the heart muscle which may arise from a number of different causes including viral infections, congenital abnormalities and chronic alcoholism.

CARDIOVASCULAR SYSTEM the heart and the whole of the circulatory system, which is divided into the *systemic* (arteries and veins of the body), and *pulmonary* (arteries and veins of the lungs). The cardio-vascular system is responsible for the transport of oxygen and nutrients to the tissues, and removing waste products and carbon dioxide from them, taking these to the organs from which they are eventually eliminated.

CAROTID ARTERY one of two large arteries in the neck which branch and provide the blood supply to the head and neck. The paired common carotid arteries arise from the AORTA on the left side of the heart and from the inominate artery on the right. These continue up on either side of the neck and branch into the internal and external carotids.

CARPUS latin for wrist, consisting of eight small bones which articulate with the ULNA and RADIUS of the forearm on one side and with the *metacarpals* (bones of the hand) on the other.

CARTILAGE a type of firm connective tissue which is pliable and forms part of the skeleton. There are three different kinds: hyaline cartilage, fibro-cartilage and elastic cartilage. *Hyaline* cartilage is found at the joints of movable bones and in the trachea, nose, bronchi and as costal cartilage joining the ribs to the breast bone. *Fibro-cartilage*, which consists of cartilage and connective tissue, is found in the intervertebral discs of the spinal column and in tendons. *Elastic* cartilage is found in the external part of the ear (pinna).

CATARACT a condition in which the lens of the eye becomes opaque, which results in a blurring of vision. It may arise from a number of different causes including injury to the eye, as a congenital condition or as a result of certain diseases such as DIABETES. However, the commonest cause is advancing age during which changes naturally take place in the lens involving the protein components.

CELL the basic building block of all life and the smallest structural unit in the body. Human body cells vary in size and function and number several billion. Each cell consists of a cell body surrounded by a membrane. The cell body consists of a substance known as cytoplasm containing various organelles, and also a nucleus. The nucleus contains the CHROMOSOMES composed of the genetic material, the DNA. Most human body cells contain 46 chromosomes (23 pairs), half being derived from the individual's father and half from the mother. Cells are able to make exact copies of themselves by a process known as MITOSIS and a full complement of chromosomes is received by each daughter cell. However, the human sex cells (sperm and ova) differ in always containing half the number of chromosomes. At fertilization, a sperm and ovum combine and a complete set of chromosomes is received by the new embryo. *See* MITOSIS and MEIOSIS.

CENTRAL NERVOUS SYSTEM the brain and the spinal cord which receives and integrates all the nervous information from the peripheral nervous system.

CEREBELLUM the largest part of the hind brain consisting of a pair of joined hemispheres. It has an outer grey cortex which is a much folded layer of grey matter and an inner core of white matter. The cerebellum co-ordinates the activity of various groups of voluntary muscles and maintains posture and balance.

CEREBRAL CORTEX the outer layer of grey matter of the cerebral hemispheres of the CEREBRUM. It is highly folded and contains many millions of nerve cells, and makes up about 40% of the brain by weight. The cerebral cortex controls intellectual processes such as thought, perception, memory and intellect, and is also involved in the senses of sight, touch and hearing. It also controls the voluntary movement of muscles and is connected with all the different parts of the body.

CEREBRUM the largest and most highly developed part of the brain consisting of a pair of cerebral hemispheres divided from each other by a longitudinal fissure. The cerebral hemispheres are covered by the CEREBRAL CORTEX below which lies white matter in which the BASAL GANGLIA are situated. The cerebrum controls complex intellectual activities and also all the voluntary responses of the body.

CERVIX a neck-like structure especially the cervix uteri or neck of the womb. It is partly above and partly within the vagina projecting into it and linking it with the cavity of the uterus via the cervical canal.

CHICKEN POX a highly infectious disease which mainly affects children and is caused by the *Varicella zoster* virus. There is an incubation period of two to three weeks and then usually a child becomes slightly feverish and unwell. Within twenty-four hours an itchy rash appears on the skin which consists of fluid-filled blisters. Eventually these form scabs which fall off after about one week. The treatment consists of the application of calamine lotion to reduce the itching, and isolation from other children.

CHILBLAIN a round, itchy inflammation of the skin which usually occurs on the toes or fingers during cold weather, and is caused by a localized deficiency in the circulation. Chilblains may sometimes be an indication of poor health or inadequate clothing and nutrition.

CHOLERA an infection of the small intestine caused by the BACTERIUM *Vibrio cholerae*. It varies in degree from very mild cases to extremely severe illness and death. During epidemics of cholera, the death rate is over 50% and these occur in conditions of poor sanitation and overcrowding. The disease is spread through con-tamination of drinking water by faeces of those affected by the disease, and also by flies landing on infected material and then crawling on food. Epidemics are rare in conditions of good sanitation but when cholera is detected, extreme attention has to be paid to hygiene including treatment and scrupulous disposal of the body waste of the infected person.

Tetracycline or other sulphonamide drugs are given to kill the bacteria. The death rate is low (5%) in those given proper and prompt treatment but the risk is greater in children and the elderly. Vaccination against cholera can be given but it is only effective for about 6 months.

CHOLESTEROL a fatty insoluble molecule (sterol) which is widely found in the body and is synthesized from saturated fatty acids in the liver. Cholesterol is an important substance in the body being a component of cell membranes and a precursor in the production of steroid hormones (sex hormones) and bile salts. An elevated level of blood cholesterol is associated with ATHEROMA which may result in high blood pressure and coronary thrombosis, and this is seen in the disease, DIABETES MELLITUS.

CHROMOSOMES the rod-like structures present in the nucleus of every body cell which carry the genetic information or genes. Each human body cell contains twenty-three pairs of chromosomes (apart from the sperm and ova), half derived from the mother and half from the father. Each chromosome consists of a coiled double filament (double helix) of DNA with genes carrying the genetic information arranged linearly along its length. The genes determine all the characteristics of each individual. Twenty-two of the pairs of chromosomes are the same in males and females. The twenty-third pair are the sex chromosomes and males have one X and one Y whereas females have two X chromosomes. *See* CELL and SEX-LINKED INHERITANCE.

CIRCULATION OF THE BLOOD the basic circulation is as follows: all the blood from the body returns to the heart via the veins, eventually entering the right atrium through the inferior and superior venae cavae.

This contracts and forces the blood into the right ventricle and from there is driven to the lungs via the pulmonary artery. In the lungs, oxygen is taken up and carbon dioxide is released and the blood then passes into the pulmonary veins and is returned to the left atrium of the heart. Blood is forced from the left atrium into the left ventricle and from there into the aorta. The aorta branches giving off the various arteries which carry the blood to all the different parts of the body. The blood eventually enters the fine network of arterioles and capillaries and supplies all the tissues and organs with oxygen and nutrients. It passes into the venules and veins, eventually returning to the right atrium through the vena cavae to complete the cycle.

CIRRHOSIS a disease of the liver in which fibrous tissue resembling scar tissue is produced as a result of damage and death to the cells. The liver becomes yellow-coloured and nodular in appearance, and there are various types of the disease including alcoholic cirrhosis and postnecrotic cirrhosis caused by viral hepatitis. The cause of the cirrhosis is not always found (cryptogenic cirrhosis) but the progress of the condition can be halted if this can be identified and removed.

CLAVICLE the collar bone forming a part of the shoulder girdle of the skeleton. It is the most commonly fractured bone in the body.

CLOT the term applied to a semi-solid lump of blood or other fluid in the body. A blood clot consists of a fine network of FIBRIN in which blood corpuscles are caught, *see* COAGULATION.

COAGULATION (of the blood) the natural process in which blood is converted from a liquid to a semi-solid state to arrest bleeding (haemorrhage). A substance known as prothrombin and calcium are

normally present in the blood, and the enzyme thromboplastin is present in the platelets (*see* BLOOD). When bleeding occurs, thromboplastin is released and prothrombin and calcium are converted by the enzyme into thrombin. A soluble protein called fibrinogen is always present in the blood and is converted by thrombin into fibrin which is the final stage in the coagulation process. A fibrous meshwork or clot is produced consisting of fibrin and blood cells which seals off the damaged blood vessel.

COCCYX the end of the backbone, which consists of four fused and reduced vertebrae which correspond to the tail of other mammals. The coccyx is surrounded by muscle and joins with the SACRUM, a further group of fused vertebrae which is part of the pelvis.

COCHLEA a spiral-shaped organ resembling a snail shell forming a part of the inner ear and concerned with hearing. It consists of three fluid-filled canals with receptors which detect pressure changes caused by sound waves. Nerve impulses are sent to the brain where the information is received and decoded.

COLD (common cold) widespread and mild infection of the upper respiratory tract caused by a virus. There is inflammation of the mucous membranes and symptoms include feverishness, coughing, sneezing, runny nose, sore throat, headache and sometimes face ache due to catarrh in the SINUSES. The disease is spread by coughing and sneezing and treatment is by means of bed rest and the taking of mild ANALGESICS.

COLD SORE *see* HERPES SIMPLEX.

COLIC spasmodic, severe abdominal pain which occurs in waves with brief interludes in between. Intestinal colic is usually the result of the presence of some indigestible food which causes the contraction of the intestinal muscles. Infantile colic, common in young babies, is due to wind associated with feeding. An attack of colic is generally not serious but can result in a twisting of the bowel which must receive immediate medical attention. Colic-type pain may also be caused by an obstruction in the bowel such as a tumour which again requires early medical treatment.

COLITIS inflammation of the colon, the symptoms of which include abdominal pain and diarrhoea, sometimes blood-stained. *Ulcerative colitis* tends to affect young adults and tends to occur periodically over a number of years. There is abdominal discomfort, fever, frequent watery diarrhoea containing mucus and blood, and anaemia. The condition can be fatal but usually there is a gradual recovery. Treatment is by means of bed rest, drug treatment with corticosteroids and iron supplements, and a bland, low roughage diet. Colitis may be due to infections caused by the organism *Entamoeba histolytica* (amoebic colitis) and by bacteria (infective colitis).

COLLAR BONE *see* CLAVICLE.

COLON the main part of the large intestine which removes water and salts from the undigested food passed into it from the small intestine. When water has been extracted the remains of the food (faeces) are passed on to the rectum.

COMA a state of deep unconsciousness from which a person cannot be roused. There may be an absence of pupillary and corneal reflexes and no movements of withdrawal when painful stimuli are applied. It may be accompanied by deep, noisy breathing and strong heart action and is caused by a number of different conditions. These include apoplexy, high fever, brain injury, diabetes

mellitus, carbon monoxide poisoning and drug overdose. A comatose person may eventually die but can recover depending upon the nature of the coma and its cause.

COMMINUTED FRACTURE a serious injury to a bone in which more than one break occurs accompanied by splintering and damage to the surrounding tissues. It usually results from a crushing force, with damage to nerves, muscles and blood vessels, and the bone is difficult to set.

COMPRESS a pad soaked in hot or cold water, wrung out and applied to an inflamed or painful part of the body. A hot compress is called a fomentation.

CONCUSSION a loss of consciousness caused by a blow to the head. The sudden knock to the head causes a compression wave which momentarily interrupts the blood supply to the brain. The unconsciousness may last for seconds or hours and when the person comes round there may be some headache and irritability which can last for some time. A mild case of concussion may not involve complete loss of consciousness but be marked by giddiness, confusion and headache. In all cases, the person needs to rest and remain under observation.

CONE a type of photoreceptor (light-sensitive cell) found in the RETINA of the eye which detects colour. Cones contain the pigment retinene and the protein opsin and there are three different types which react to light of differing wavelengths, (blue, green and red).

CONGENITAL diseases or conditions that are present at birth.

CONJUNCTIVITIS inflammation of the mucous membrane (conjunctiva) that lines the inside of the eyelid and covers the front of the eye. The eyes become pink and watery and the condition is usually caused by an infection which may be bacterial, viral or the micro-organism *Chlamydia* may be responsible. Treatment depends upon cause but a number of drugs are used often in the form of eyedrops.

CONNECTIVE TISSUE supporting or packing tissue within the body which holds or separates other tissues and organs. It consists of a ground material composed of substances called muco-polysaccharides. In this, certain fibres such as yellow elastic, white collagenous and reticular fibres are embedded along with a variety of other cells, e.g MAST CELLS, MACROPHAGES, fibroblasts and fat cells. The constituents vary in proportions in different kinds of connective tissue to produce a number of distinct types. Examples are adipose (fatty) tissue, cartilage, bone, tends and ligaments.

CONSTIPATION the condition in which the bowels are opened too infrequently and the faeces become dry, hard and difficult and painful to pass. The frequency of normal bowel opening varies between people but when constipation becomes a problem, it is usually a result of inattention to this habit or to the diet. To correct the condition a change of lifestyle may be needed including taking more exercise, fluid and roughage in the diet. Laxatives and enemas are also used to alleviate the condition. Constipation is also a symptom of the more serious condition of blockage of the bowel (by a tumour), but this is less common.

CONTROLLED DRUGS those drugs which, in the United Kingdom, are subject to the restrictions of the Misuse of Drugs Act 1971. They are classified into three categories: Class A includes LSD, morphine, cocaine and pethidine. Class B includes

cannabis, amphetamines and barbiturates and Class C comprises amphetamine-related drugs and some others.

CONVULSIONS also known as fits, these are involuntary, alternate, rapid, muscular contractions and relaxations throwing the body and limbs into contortions. They are caused by a disturbance of brain function and in adults usually result from epilepsy. In babies and young children they occur quite commonly but, although alarming, are generally not serious. Causes include a high fever due to infection, brain diseases such as meningitis and breath-holding, which is quite common in infants and very young children. Convulsions are thought to be more common in the very young because the nervous system is immature. Unless they are caused by the presence of disease or infection which requires to be treated, they are rarely life-threatening.

CORNEA the outermost, exposed layer of the EYE which is transparent and lies over the iris and lens. It refracts light entering the eye, directing the rays to the lens and thus acting as a coarse focus. It is a layer of connective tissue which has no blood supply of its own but is supplied with nutrients from fluid within the eye (the aqueous humour). It is highly sensitive to pain and presence or absence of response if the cornea is touched is used as an indicator of a person's condition, for example in a comatose patient.

CORONARY ARTERIES the arteries that supply blood to the heart and which arise from the AORTA.

CORONARY ARTERY DISEASE any abnormal condition that affects the arteries of the heart. The commonest disease is coronary ATHEROSCLEROSIS which is more prevalent in those populations with high fat, saturated fat, refined

carbohydrates etc. in their diet.
ANGINA is a common symptom of
such diseases.

CORONARY THROMBOSIS a
sudden blockage of one of the
coronary arteries by a blood clot or
thrombus which interrupts the blood
supply to the heart. The victim
collapses with severe and agonizing
chest pain often accompanied by
vomiting and nausea. The skin
becomes pale and clammy, the
temperature rises and there is
difficulty in breathing. Coronary
thrombosis generally results from
ATHEROMA, and the part of the heart
muscle which has its blood supply
disrupted dies, a condition known as
MYOCARDIAL INFARCTION. Treatment
consists of giving strong pain-
relieving drugs such as morphine.
Also specialist care in a coronary
care unit is usually required to deal
with ARRHYTHMIA, heart failure and
CARDIAC ARREST which are the
potentially fatal results of coronary
thrombosis.

COT DEATH see SUDDEN INFANT
DEATH SYNDROME.

CRAMP prolonged and painful
spasmodic muscular contraction
which often occurs in the limbs but
can affect certain internal organs
(see COLIC and GASTRALGIA). Cramp
may result from a salt imbalance as
in heat cramp. Working in high
temperatures causes excessive
sweating and consequent loss of salt.
It can be corrected and prevented by
an increase of the salt intake.
Occupational cramp results from
continual repetitive use of particular
muscles, e.g. writer's cramp. Night
cramp occurs during sleep and is
especially common among elderly
people, diabetics and pregnant
women. The cause of night cramp is
not known.

CRANIUM the part of the skull that
encloses the brain, formed from
eight fused and flattened bones that
are joined by immovable suture
JOINTS.

CROUP a group of diseases
characterized by a swelling, partial
obstruction and inflammation of the
entrance to the larynx, occurring in
young children. The breathing is
harsh and strained producing a
typical crowing sound, accompanied
by coughing and feverishness.
Diphtheria used to be the most
common cause of croup but it now
usually results from a viral infection
of the respiratory tract (LARYNGO-
TRACHEO BRONCHITIS). The condition
is relieved by inhaling steam (a
soothing preparation such as tincture
of benzoin is sometimes added to the
hot water) and also by mild sedatives
and/or pain killers. Rarely, the
obstruction becomes dangerous and
completely blocks the larynx in
which case emergency TRACHEOSTO-
MY or nasotracheal INTUBATION may
be required.

CYANOSIS a blue appearance of
the skin due to insufficient oxygen
within the blood. It is first noticeable
on the lips, tips of the ears, cheeks and
nails and occurs in heart failure, lung
diseases, asphyxia and in 'blue babies'
who have congenital heart defects.

CYSTS small, usually benign,
tumours containing fluid (or soft
secretions) within a membranous
sac. Examples are wens (caused by
blockage of sebaceous glands in the
skin), cysts in the breasts caused by
blocked milk ducts and ovarian cysts
which may be large and contain a
clear, thick liquid.

D

DEFIBRILLATION the application
of a large electric shock to the chest
wall of a patient whose heart is
fibrillating (see FIBRILLATION). The

delivery of a direct electric countershock hopefully allows the pacemaker to set up the correct rhythm again.

DEHYDRATION the removal of water. More specifically, the loss of water from the body through diuresis, sweating etc. or a reduction in water content due to a low intake. Essential body electrolytes (such as sodium chloride and potassium) are disrupted and after the first symptom, thirst, irritability and confusion follow.

DELIRIUM a mental disorder typified by confusion, agitation, fear, anxiety, illusions and sometimes hallucinations. The causal cerebral disfunction may be due to deficient nutrition, stress, toxic poisoning or mental shock.

DERMATITIS an inflammation of the skin which is similar in many respects to, and often interchanged with, ECZEMA. It is characterized by erythema (redness due to dilatation of capillaries near the surface), pain and PRURITIS. Several forms of dermatitis can be identified: Contact dermatitis, light dermatitis and erythroderma, which is often associated with other skin conditions, e.g. PSORIASIS.

DIABETES INSIPIDUS a rare condition which is completely different from DIABETES MELLITUS and is characterized by excessive thirst (see POLYDIPSIA) and POLYURIA. It is due to a lack of the antidiuretic hormone or the inability of the kidney to respond to the hormone.

DIABETES MELLITUS a complex metabolic disorder involving carbohydrate, fat and protein. It results in an accumulation of sugar in the blood and urine and is due to a lack of INSULIN produced by the pancreas, so that sugars are not broken down to release energy. Fats are thus used as an alternative energy source. Symptoms include

thirst, POLYURIA, loss of weight and the use of fats can produce KETOSIS and KETONURIA. In its severest form, convulsions are followed by a diabetic coma.

Treatment relies upon dietary control with doses of insulin or drugs, long-term effects include thickening of the arteries, and in some cases the eyes, kidneys, nervous system, skin and circulation may be affected (see also HYPOGLYCAEMIA and HYPERGLY-CAEMIA).

DIALYSIS the use of a semiper-meable membrane to separate large and small molecules by selective diffusion. Starch and proteins are large molecules while salts, glucose and amino acids are small molecules. If a mixture of large and small molecules is separated from distilled water by a semi-permeable membrane, the smaller molecules diffuse into the water which is itself replenished. This principle is the basis of the artificial kidney which, because a patient's blood is processed, is known as haemodialy-sis.

DIAPHRAGM a membrane of muscle and tendon that separates the thoracic and abdominal cavities. It is covered by a SEROUS MEMBRANE and attached at the lower ribs, breastbone and backbone. The diaphragm is important in breathing, when it bulges up to its resting position during exhalation. It flattens during inhalation and in so doing it reduces pressure in the thoracic cavity and helps to draw air into the lungs.

DIAPHYSIS the central part of shaft of a long bone.

DIARRHOEA increased frequency and looseness of bowel movement, involving the passage of unusually soft faeces. Diarrhoea can be caused by food poisoning, COLITIS, IRRITABLE BOWEL SYNDROME, DYSENTERY, etc. A severe case will result in the loss of water and salts which must be replaced and anti-diarrhoeal drugs are used in certain circumstances.

DIASTOLE the point at which the heart relaxes between contractions, when the ventricles fill with blood. This usually lasts about half a second at the end of which the ventricles are about three-quarters full.

DIGESTION the process of breaking down food into substances that can be absorbed and used by the body. Digestion begins with the chewing and grinding of food at which point it is mixed with saliva to commence the process of break-down. Most digestion occurs in the stomach and small intestine. In the stomach the food is subject to gastric juice which contains pepsins to break down proteins and hydrochloric acid. The food is mixed and becomes totally soluble before passing into the small intestine as chyme, where it is acted upon by pancreatic juice, bile, bacteria and *succus entericus* (intestinal juices).

Water is absorbed in the intestine in a very short time, while the bulk of the food may take several hours. The chyme forms chyle due to the action of bile and pancreatic juice. Fats are removed from this in emulsion form into the lymph vessels (*see* LACTEAL) and then into the blood. Sugars, salts and amino acids move directly into the small blood vessels in the intestine and the whole process is promoted by microfolding of the intestine wall producing finger-like projections (villi). The food passes down the intestine due to muscle contractions of the intestine wall and ultimately the residue and waste are excreted.

DIPLEGIA paralysis on both sides of the body.

DIPLOPIA double vision. Caused by dysfunction in the muscles that move the eyeballs such that rays of light fall in different places on the two retinae. The condition can be due to a nervous disease, intoxication or certain diseases such as diphtheria.

DISC a flattened circular structure, such as the cartilage between vertebrae.

DISINFECTION the process of killing PATHOGENIC organisms (not spores) to prevent the spread of infection. Different compounds are used, appropriate to the surface being disinfected.

DIURESIS an increase in urine production due to disease, drugs, hormone imbalance or increased fluid intake.

DIVERTICULUM in general, a pouch extending from a main cavity. Specifically applied to the intestine, a sac-like protrusion through the wall, many of which usually develop later in life and is thought to be related to dietary factors. The formation of diverticula is diverticulosis and their inflammation (causing pain, pyrexia and constipation), diverticulitis.

DUCT a narrow tube-like structure joining a gland with an organ or the body surface, through which a secretion passes e.g. sweat ducts opening onto the skin.

DUODENAL ULCER the commonest type of PEPTIC ULCER. Duodenal ulcers may occur after the age of 20 and are more common in men. The cause is open to debate but probably results from an abrasion or break in the duodenum lining which is then exacerbated by gastric juice. Smoking seems to be a contributory but not a causal factor.

The ulcer manifests itself as an upper abdominal pain roughly two hours after a meal that also occurs during the night. Food (e.g. milk) relieves the symptom and a regime of frequent meals and milky snacks, with little or no fried food and spices and a minimum of strong tea and coffee is usually adopted. Recent drug treatments enable the acid secretion to be reduced, thus allowing the ulcer to heal. Surgery is required only if there is no response to treatment, if the pylorus is obstructed or if the ulcer becomes perforated. The latter is treated as an emergency.

DUODENUM the first part of the small intestine where food (chyme) from the stomach is subject to action by BILE and pancreatic enzymes. The duodenum also secretes a hormone secretion that contributes to the breakdown of fats, proteins and carbohydrates. In the duodenum, the acid conditions pertaining from the stomach are neutralized and rendered alkaline for the intestinal enzymes to operate.

DURA MATER *see* MENINGES and BRAIN.

DYSENTERY an infection and ulceration of the lower part of the bowels that causes severe diarrhoea with the passage of mucus and blood. There are two forms of dysentery caused by different organisms. Amoebic dysentery is due to *Entamoeba histolytica* which is spread via infected food or water and occurs mainly in the tropics and sub-tropics. The appearance of symptoms may be delayed but in addition to diarrhoea there is indigestion, anaemia and weight loss. Drugs are used in treatment.

Bacillary dysentery is caused by the bacterium *Shigella* and spreads by contact with a carrier or contaminated food. Symptoms appear from one to six days after infection and include diarrhoea, cramp, nausea, fever and the severity of the attack varies.

DYSPEPSIA (or indigestion) after eating there may be discomfort in the upper abdomen/lower chest with heartburn, nausea and flatulence accompanying a feeling of fullness. The causes are numerous and include GALLSTONES, PEPTIC ULCER,

HIATUS HERNIA and diseases of the liver or pancreas.

DYSPHASIA a general term for an impairment of speech whether it is manifested as a difficulty in understanding language or in self-expression. There is a range of conditions with varying degrees of severity. *Global aphasia* is a total inability to communicate, however some individuals partially understand what is said to them. *Dysphasia* is when thoughts can be expressed up to a point. *Non-fluent dysphasia* represents poor self-expression but good understanding while the reverse is called *fluent dysphasia*. The condition may be due to a stroke or other brain damage and can be temporary or permanent.

E

EAR the sense organ used for detection of sound and maintenance of balance. It comprises three parts, the external or outer, middle and inner ear, the first two acting to collect sound waves and transmit them to the inner ear, where the hearing and balance mechanisms are situated. The outer ear (*auricle* or *pinna*) is a cartilage and skin structure which is not actually essential to hearing in man. The middle ear is an air-filled cavity that is linked to the PHARYNX via the EUSTACHIAN TUBE. Within the middle ear are the ear (or auditory) ossicles, three bones called the *incus, malleus* and *stapes* (anvil, hammer and stirrup respectively). Two small muscles control the bones and the associated nerve (the chorda tympani). The ossicles bridge the middle ear, connecting the eardrum with the inner ear and in so doing convert sound (air waves) into mechanical movements which then impinge upon the fluid of the inner ear.

The inner ear lies within the temporal bone of the skull and contains the apparatus for hearing and balance. The COCHLEA is responsible for hearing and balance is maintained by the semi-circular canals. The latter are made up of three loops positioned mutually at right angles and in each is the fluid endolymph. When the head is moved the fluid moves accordingly and sensory cells produce impulses that are transmitted to the brain.

EARACHE pain in the ear may be due directly to inflammation of the middle ear but is often referred pain from other conditions, e.g. infections of the nose, larynx or tooth decay.

ECLAMPSIA convulsions that occur during pregnancy, usually at the later stages or during delivery. Although the cause is not known the start of convulsions may be associated with cerebral OEDEMA or a sudden rise in blood pressure. Kidney function is usually badly affected. The condition is often preceded for days or weeks by symptoms such as headache, dizziness and vomiting and seizures follow. The fits differ in severity and duration and in the one in twelve fatalities, there may be a cerebral haemorrhage, pneumonia or the breathing may gradually fade. The condition requires immediate treatment as it threatens both mother and baby. Treatment is by drugs and reduction of outside stimuli, and a CAESARIAN SECTION is undertaken.

ECZEMA an inflammation of the skin that causes itching, a red rash and often small blisters that weep and become encrusted. This may be followed by the skin thickening and then peeling off in scales. There are several types of eczema, *atopic* being one of the most common. (Atopic is the hereditary tendency to form allergic reactions due to an

antibody in the skin). A form of atopic eczema is infantile eczema that starts at 3 or 4 months and it is often the case that eczema, hay fever and asthma is found in the family history. However, many children improve markedly as they approach the age of 10 or 11. The treatment for such conditions usually involves the use of HYDROCORTISONE and other steroid creams and ointments.

ELECTROLYTES *sensu stricto* - a compound that dissolves in water to produce a solution containing ions that is able to conduct an electrical charge. In the body, electrolytes occur in the blood plasma, all fluid and interstitial fluid and normal concentrations are imperative for normal metabolic activity. Some diseases alter the electrolyte balance either through vomiting or diarrhoea or because the kidney is malfunctioning. The correct balance can be restored through oral or intravenous dosage or by DIALYSIS.

EMBOLISM the state in which a small blood vessel is blocked by an EMBOLUS, or fragment of material which the circulatory system has carried through larger vessels. This plug may be fragments of a clot, a mass of bacteria, air bubbles that have entered the system during an operation, or a fragment of tumour. The blockage leads usually to the destruction of that part of the organ supplied by the vessel. The most common case is a pulmonary embolism. Treatment utilises an anticoagulant drug such as warfarin or heparin, embolectomy or streptokinase.

EMBOLUS material carried by the blood which then lodges elsewhere in the body (*see* EMBOLISM). The material may be a blood clot, fat, air, a piece of tumour etc.

EMESIS is the medical term for vomit.

EMPHYSEMA refers, in the main,

to an abnormal condition of the lungs where the walls of the alveoli are over-inflated and distended and changes in their structure occur. This destruction of parts of the walls produces large air-filled spaces which do not contribute to the respiratory process. Acute cases of emphysema may be caused by whooping cough, bronchopneumonia and chronic cases often accompany chronic bronchitis which itself is due in great part to smoking. Emphysema is also developed after tuberculosis when the lungs are stretched until the fibres of the alveolar walls are destroyed. Similarly in old age, the alveolar membrane may collapse producing large air sacs, with decreased surface area.

ENCEPHALITIS inflammation of the brain. It is usually a viral infection and sometimes occurs as a complication of some common infectious diseases, e.g. measles or chickenpox. There are several forms of the disease including *Encephalitis lethargica* (sleepy sickness or epidemic encephalitis) which attacks and causes swelling in the basal ganglia, cerebrum and brain stem that may result in tissue destruction.

ENCEPHALOMYELITIS inflammation of the brain and spinal cord typified by headaches, fever, stiff neck and back pain, with vomiting. Depending upon the extent of the inflammation and the patient's condition, encephalomyelitis may cause paralysis, personality changes, coma or death.

ENCEPHALOPATHY any disease affecting the brain or an abnormal condition of the brain's structure and function. It refers in particular to degenerative and chronic conditions such as Wernicke's encephalopathy which is caused by a thiamine deficiency and associated with alcoholism.

ENDEMIC the term used to describe, for example, a disease that is indigenous to a certain area.

ENDOCARDIUM a fine membrane lining the heart which forms a continuous membrane with the lining of veins and arteries. At the cavities of the heart it forms cusps on the valves and its surface is very smooth to facilitate blood flow.

ENDOCRINE GLANDS DUCTLESS GLANDS that produce HORMONES for secretion directly into the bloodstream (or lymph). Some organs e.g. the PANCREAS also release secretions via a DUCT. In addition to the pancreas the major endocrine glands are the THYROID, PITUITARY, PARATHYROID, OVARY and TESTIS. Imbalances in the secretions of endocrine glands produce a variety of diseases (*see individual entries*).

ENDOGENOUS referring to within the body, whether growing within, or originating from within or due to internal causes.

ENTERITIS inflammation of the intestine, due usually to a viral or bacterial infection, causing diarrhoea.

ENZYME any protein molecule that acts as a catalyst in the biochemical processes of the body. They are essential to life and are highly specific, acting on certain substrates at a set temperature and pH. Examples are the digestive enzymes amylase, lipase and trypsin. Enzymes act by providing active sites (one or more for each enzyme) to which substrate molecules bind, forming a short-lived intermediate. The rate of reaction is increased, and after the product is formed, the active site is freed. Enzymes are easily rendered inactive by heat and some chemicals. Enzymes are vital for the normal functioning of the body and their lack or inactivity can produce metabolic disorders.

EPIDEMIC a disease that affects a

large proportion of the population at the same time. Usually an infectious disease that occurs suddenly and spreads rapidly, e.g. today there are influenza epidemics.

EPIDERMIS the outer layer of the skin which comprises four layers and overlies the dermis. The top three layers are continually renewed as cells from the innermost germinative layer (called *the Malpighian layer or stratum germinativum*) are pushed outwards. The topmost layer (*stratum corneum*) is made up of dead cells where the CYTOPLASM has been replaced by KERATIN. This layer is thickest on the palms and soles of the feet.

EPIGLOTTIS situated at the base of the tongue, a thin piece of cartilage enclosed in MUCOUS MEMBRANE that covers the LARYNX. It prevents food from passing into the larynx and TRACHEA when swallowing. The epiglottis resembles a leaf in shape.

EPIGLOTTITIS inflammation of the mucous membrane of the EPIGLOTTIS. Swelling of the tissues may obstruct the airway and swift action may be necessary i.e. a TRACHEOSTOMY to avoid a fatality. The other symptoms of epiglottitis are sore throat, fever, a croup-like cough and it occurs mainly in children, usually during the winter.

EPILEPSY a neurological disorder involving convulsions, seizures and loss of consciousness. There are many possible causes or associations of epilepsy, including cerebral trauma, brain tumour, cerebral haemorrhage and metabolic imbalances as in HYPOGLYCAEMIA. Usually an epileptic attack occurs without warning, with complete unconsciousness and some muscle contraction and spasms. Some drugs are used in treatment although little can be done during the fit itself.

EPIPHYSIS the softer end of a long

bone that is separated from the shaft by a plate (the epiphyseal plate) of cartilage. It develops separately from the shaft but when the bone stops growing it disappears as the head and shaft fuse. Separation of the epiphysis is a serious fracture because the growing bone may be affected.

EPITHELIUM (*plural* **EPITHE-LIA**) tissue made up of cells packed closely together and bound by connective material. It covers the outer surface of the body and lines vessels and organs in the body. One surface is fixed to a basement membrane and the other is free and it provides a barrier against injury, micro-organisms and some fluid loss. There are various types of epithelium in single and multiple (or stratified) layers and differing shapes *viz.* cuboidal, squamous (like flat pads) and columnar.

ERUPTION an outbreak, or rash upon the skin usually in the form of a red and raised area, possibly with fluid-containing vesicles or scales/crusts. It may be associated with a disease such as measles or chickenpox, a drug reaction or a physical or short-lived occurrence, e.g. nettle-rash.

ERYTHEMA an inflammation or redness of the skin in which the tissues are congested with blood. The condition may be accompanied by pain or itching. There are numerous causes, some bacterial/viral and others physical e.g. mild sunburn.

ERYTHROCYTE the red blood cell that is made in the bone marrow and occurs as a red disc, concave on both sides, full of HAEMOGLOBIN. These cells are responsible for carrying oxygen to tissues and carbon dioxide away The latter is removed in the form of the bicarbonate ion (HCO_3^-), in exchange for a chloride ion (Cl^-).

ESCHERICHIA a group of gram-negative (*see* GRAM'S STAIN) rod-shaped bacteria (*E. coli*) normally found in the intestines and common in water, milk etc. *E. coli* is a common cause of infections of the urinary tract.

ESSENTIAL HYPERTENSION high blood pressure with no identifiable cause. Arteriosclerosis is a complication of, and often associated with hypertension. Other complications include cerebral haemorrhage, heart failure and kidney failure. There are now several drugs that reduce blood pressure, including beta-blockers and methyldopa. Lifestyle is an important factor for some sufferers: excessive weight should be lost, excess salt intake avoided and strain of all types lessened.

EUSTACHIAN TUBE tubes, one on each side, that connect the middle ear to the PHARYNX. The short (about 35–40mm) tube is fine at the centre and wider at both ends and is lined with mucous membrane. It is normally closed but opens to equalize air pressure on either side of the eardrum.

EXCORIATION injury of the surface of the skin (or other part of the body) caused by the abrasion or scratching of the area.

EXCRETION the removal of all waste material (excreta) from the body, including urine and faeces, the loss of water and salts through sweat glands, and the elimination of carbon dioxide and water vapour from the lungs.

EXOGENOUS originating outside the body, and can also refer to an organ of the body.

EXTRASYSTOLE (*or* ECTOPIC BEAT) a heart beat that is outside the normal rhythm of the heart and is due to an impulse generated outside the SINOATRIAL NODE. It may go unnoticed or it may seem that the heart has missed a beat. Extrasystoles are common in healthy people,

but they may result from heart disease, or nicotine from smoking, or caffeine from excessive intake of tea and coffee. Drugs can be taken to suppress these irregular beats.

EYE the complicated organ of sight. Each eye is roughly spherical and contained within the bony ORBIT in the skull. The outer layer is fibrous and comprises the opaque SCLERA and transparent CORNEA. The middle layer is vascular and is made up of the *choroid* (the blood supply for the outer half of the retina), *ciliary body* (which secretes aqueous humour) and the IRIS. The inner layer is sensory, the RETINA. Between the cornea and the LENS is a chamber filled with aqueous humour and behind the lens is a much larger cavity with vitreous humour. Light enters the eye through the cornea and thence via the aqueous humour to the lens which focuses the light onto the retina. The latter contains CONE and ROD cells which are sensitive to light and impulses are sent to the visual cortex of the brain via the optic nerve.

F

FACE the front-facing part of the head which extends from the chin to the forehead. There are fourteen bones in the skull, supporting the face, and numerous fine muscles are responsible for movements around the eyes, nose and mouth producing expression. These are under the control of the 7th cranial nerve which is a mixed sensory and motor nerve known as the FACIAL NERVE.

FACIAL NERVE the cranial nerve which has a number of branches and supplies the muscles which control facial expression. It also has branches to the middle ear, taste buds, salivary glands and lacrimal glands. Some branches are motor and others sensory in function.

FACIAL PARALYSIS paralysis of the facial nerve, which leads to a loss of function in the muscles of the face producing a lack of expression in the affected side. It occurs in the condition known as *Bell's palsy* in which there may also be a loss of taste and inability to close the eye. The condition is often temporary, if caused by inflammation which recovers in time. However, if the nerve itself is damaged by injury or if the person has suffered a stroke, the condition is likely to be permanent.

FAECES the end waste product of digestion which is formed in the colon and discharged from the bowels via the ANUS. Also known as stools, it consists of undigested food (chiefly cellulose), bacteria, mucus and other secretions, water and bile pigments which are responsible for the colour. The condition and colour of the faeces are indicators of general health e.g. pale stools are produced in JAUNDICE and COELIAC DISEASE and black stools often indicate the presence of digested blood.

FALLOPIAN TUBES a pair of tubes, one of which leads from each ovary to the womb. At the ovary, the tube is expanded to form a funnel with finger-like projections, known as fimbriae, surrounding the opening. This funnel does not communicate directly with the ovary but is open to the abdominal cavity. However, when an egg is released from the ovary the fimbriae move and waft it into the fallopian tube. The tube is about 10 to 12cm long and leads directly in to the womb at the lower end through a narrow opening.

FAT *see* ADIPOSE TISSUE.

FEBRILE having a fever.

FEMORAL describing the femur or area of the thigh e.g. femoral artery, vein, nerve and canal.

FEMUR the thigh bone which is the long bone extending from the hip to the knee and is the strongest bone in the body. It is the weight-bearing bone of the body and fractures are common in old people who have lost bone mass. It articulates with the pelvic girdle at the upper end, forming the hip joint and at the lower end with the patella (knee cap) and tibia to form the knee joint.

FERTILIZATION the fusion of SPERM (-ATOZOON) and OVUM to form a *zygote* which then undergoes cell division to become an embryo. Fertilization in humans takes place high up in the FALLOPIAN TUBE near the ovary and the fertilized egg travels down and becomes implanted in the womb.

FEVER an elevation of body temperature above the normal which accompanies many diseases and infections. The cause of fever is the production by the body of endogenous pyrogen which acts on the thermo-regulatory centre in the hypothalamus of the brain. This responds by promoting mechanisms which increase heat generation and lessen heat loss, leading to a rise in temperature. Fever is the main factor in many infections caused by bacteria or viruses and results from toxins produced by the growth of these organisms. An *intermittent fever* describes a fluctuating body temperature, in which the temperature sometimes returns to normal. In a *remittent fever* there is also a fluctuating body temperature but this does not return to normal. In a *relapsing fever*, caused by bacteria of the genus *Borella*, transmitted by ticks or lice, there is a recurrent fever every 3 to 10 days following the first attack which lasts for about one week.

Treatment of fever depends upon the underlying cause. However, it may be necessary to reduce the temperature by direct methods such as sponging the body with tepid water, or by giving drugs such as ASPIRIN. As well as a rise in body temperature, symptoms of fever include headache, shivering, nausea, diarrhoea or constipation. Above 105°F, there may be delirium or convulsions, especially in young children.

FIBRILLATION The rapid non-synchronized contraction or tremor of muscles in which individual bundles of fibres contract independently. It applies especially to heart muscle and disrupts the normal beating so that the affected part is unable to pump blood. Two types of fibrillation may occur depending upon which muscle is affected. Atrial fibrillation, often resulting from ATHEROSCLEROSIS or rheumatic heart disease, affects the muscles of the atria and is a common type of arrhythmia. The heart beat and pulse are very irregular and cardiac output is maintained by the contraction of the ventricles alone. With ventricular fibrillation the heart stops pumping blood so that this, in effect, is cardiac arrest. The patient requires immediate emergency resuscitation or death ensues within minutes.

FIBROID a type of benign tumour found in the womb (uterus) composed of fibrous and muscular tissue and varying in size from one or two mm to a mass weighing several pounds. They more commonly occur in childless women and those over the age of thirty five. Fibroids may present no problems but alternatively can be the cause of pain, heavy and irregular menstrual bleeding, urine retention or frequency of MICTURITION and sterility. Fibroids can be removed surgically but often the complete removal of the womb (hysterectomy)

is carried out.

FIBROMA a benign tumour composed of fibrous tissue.

FIBROSIS the formation of thickened connective or scar tissue usually as a result of injury or inflammation. This may affect the lining of the ALVEOLI of the lungs (pulmonary interstitial fibrosis) and causes breathlessness.

FIBROSITIS inflammation of fibrous connective tissue, muscles and muscle sheaths, particularly in the back, legs and arms causing pain and stiffness.

FIBROUS TISSUE a tissue type which occurs abundantly throughout the body. *White fibrous tissue* consists of collagen fibres, a protein with a high tensile strength and unyielding structure, that forms ligaments, sinews and scar tissue, and occurs in the skin. *Yellow fibrous tissue* is composed of the fibres of another protein, elastin. It is very elastic and occurs in ligaments which are subjected to frequent stretching, such as those in the back of the neck. It also occurs in arterial walls and in the walls of the alveoli (*see* ALVEOLUS), and in the dermis layer of the skin.

FIBULA the outer, thin, long bone which articulates with the larger tibia in the lower leg.

FISSURE a natural cleft or groove or abnormal break in the skin or mucous membrane e.g. an anal fissure.

FISTULA an abnormal opening between two hollow organs or between such an organ or gland and the exterior. These may arise during development so that a baby may be born with a fistula. Alternatively, they can be produced by injury, infection or as a complication following surgery. A common example is an anal fistula, which may develop if an abscess present in the rectum bursts and produces a communication through the surface of the skin.

FIT any sudden convulsive attack; a general term which is applied to an epileptic seizure, convulsion or bout of coughing.

FLATULENCE a build-up of gas in the stomach or bowels which is released through the mouth or anus.

FLEXOR any muscle that causes a limb or other body part to bend.

FLUTTER an abnormal disturbance of heart beat rhythm which may affect the atria or ventricles but is less severe than FIBRILLATION. The causes are the same as those of fibrillation and the treatment is also similar.

FLUX an excessive and abnormal flow from any of the natural openings of the body e.g. alvine flux which is diarrhoea.

FOETUS an unborn child after the eighth week of development.

FOLLICLE any small sac, cavity or secretory gland. Examples are hair follicles and the Graafian follicles of the ovaries in and from which eggs mature and are released.

FONTANELLE openings in the skull of newborn and young infants in whom the bone is not wholly formed and the sutures are incompletely fused. The largest of these is the *anterior fontanelle* on the top of the head which is about 2.5cm square at birth.

The fontanelles gradually close as bone is formed and are completely covered by the age of 18 months. If a baby is unwell, for example with a fever, the fontanelle becomes tense. If an infant is suffering from diarrhoea and possibly dehydrated, the fontanelle is abnormally depressed.

FOOD POISONING an illness of the digestive system caused by eating food contaminated by certain bacteria, viruses or by chemical poisons (insecticides) and metallic elements such as mercury or lead. Symptoms include vomiting, diarrhoea, nausea and abdominal pain and these may arise very quickly and usually within 24 hours. Bacteria are the usual cause of food poisoning and proliferate rapidly producing toxins which cause the symptoms of the illness. Those involved include members of the genera *Salmonella, Staphylococcus, Campylobacter* and also *Clostridium botulinum*, the causal organism of botulism. Food poisoning may be fatal, the old and the young being especially at risk.

FORAMEN a hole or opening which usually refers to those which occur in some bones. For example the *foramen magnum* is a large hole at the base of the skull (in the *occipital bone*) through which the spinal cord passes out from the brain.

FOSSA a natural hollow or depression on the surface or within the body. Examples include the fossae within the skull which house different parts of the brain and the cubital fossa, a hollow at the front of the elbow joint.

FRACTURE any break in a bone which may be complete or incomplete. In a *simple fracture* (or *closed fracture*) the skin remains more or less intact but in a *compound fracture* (or *open fracture*) there is an open wound connecting the bone with the surface. This type of fracture is more serious as it provides a greater risk of infection and more blood loss. If a bone which is already diseased suffers a fracture, (such as often occurs in older women who have OSTEOPOROSIS), this is known as a *pathological fracture*. A *fatigue fracture* occurs in a bone which suffers recurrent, persistent stress, e.g. the *March fracture* sometimes seen in the second toe of soldiers after long marches.

A *greenstick fracture* only occurs in young children whose bones are still soft and tend to bend. The fracture occurs on the opposite side from the causal force. A *complicated fracture* involves damage to surrounding soft tissue including nerves and blood vessels. A *depressed fracture* refers only to the skull when a piece of bone is forced inwards and may damage the brain. *See also* COMMINUTED FRACTURE.

FRONTAL LOBE the anterior part of the *cerebral hemisphere* of the CEREBRUM of the brain, extending back to a region called the central sulcus which is a deep cleft on the upper, outer surface.

FROZEN SHOULDER painful stiffness of the shoulder joint which limits movement and is more common in older people between the ages of 50 and 70. It may result from injury but often there is no apparent cause. Treatment involves exercises and sometimes injections of corticosteroid drugs, and usually there is a gradual recovery.

FUNDUS the enlarged base of an organ farthest away from its opening or a point in the RETINA of the EYE opposite the pupil.

FUNGAL DISEASES diseases or infections caused by fungi.

G

GALL another term for BILE.

GALL BLADDER a sac-like organ situated on the underside of the liver which stores and concentrates BILE. It is approximately 8cm long and 2.5cm at its widest and its volume is a little over 30cm³. When fats are digested, the gall bladder contracts, sending bile into the DUODENUM through the common bile duct. GALLSTONES, the most common gall

bladder disease, may form in certain circumstances.

GALLSTONES stones of varying composition, that form in the GALL BLADDER. Their formation seems to be due to a change in bile composition rendering cholesterol less soluble. Stones may also form around a foreign body. There are three types of stone: cholesterol, pigment and mixed, the latter being the most common. Calcium salts are usually found in varying proportions. Although gallstones may be present for years without symptoms, they can cause severe pain and may pass into the common bile duct to cause, by the resulting obstruction, jaundice.

GAMETE a mature germ or sexual cell, male or female, that can participate in fertilization e.g. OVUM and SPERMATOZOON.

GANGLION (*plural* **GANGLIA**)
1. a mass of nervous tissue containing nerve cells and SYNAPSES. Chains of ganglia are situated on each side of the spinal cord while other ganglia are sited near to or in the appropriate organs. Within the central nervous system some well-defined masses of nerve cells are called ganglia e.g. basal ganglia (*see* BASAL GANGLION).
2. a benign swelling that often forms in the sheath of a tendon and is fluid-filled. It occurs particularly at the wrist, and may disappear quite suddenly.

GANGRENE death of tissue due to loss of blood supply or bacterial infection. There are two types of gangrene, *dry* and *moist*. Dry gangrene is caused purely by loss of blood supply and is a late stage complication of DIABETES MELLITUS in which ATHEROSCLEROSIS is present. The affected part becomes cold and turns brown and black and there is an obvious line between living and dead tissue. In time the gangrenous part drops off.

GAS GANGRENE a form of gangrene that occurs when wounds are infected with soil bacteria of the genus *Clostridium*. The bacterium produces toxins that cause decay and putrefaction with the generation of gas.The gas spreads into muscles and connective tissue causing swelling, pain, fever and possibly toxic delirium, and if untreated the condition quickly leads to death. Some of these bacteria are anaerobic (exist without air or oxygen) hence surgery, oxidizing agents and penicillin can all be used in treatment.

GASTRALGIA term meaning pain in the stomach.

GASTRIC anything relating to the stomach.

GASTRIC JUICE the secretion from the gastric glands in the stomach. The main constituents are hydrochloric acid, rennin, mucin and pepsinogen, the latter forming pepsin in the acid conditions. The acidity (which is around pH 1 to 1.5) also destroys unwanted bacteria.

GASTRIC ULCER an erosion of the stomach MUCOSA caused by such agents as acid and bile. It may penetrate the muscle and perforate the stomach wall (*see* PERFORATION). Typical symptoms include burning pain, belching and possibly nausea when the stomach is empty or soon after eating. Relief may be found with antacid compounds, but surgery may be necessary.

GASTRITIS inflammation of the stomach lining (MUCOSA). It may be due to bacteria or excessive alcohol intake.

GASTROENTERITIS inflammation of both the stomach and intestines leading to vomiting and diarrhoea. It is most commonly due to viral or bacterial infection and fluid loss can be serious in children.

GENE the fundamental unit of genetic material found at a specific location on a CHROMOSOME. It is chemically complex and responsible for the transmission of information between older and younger generations. Each gene contributes to a particular trait or characteristic. There are more than 100,000 genes in man and gene size varies with the characteristic e.g. the gene that codes for the hormone INSULIN is 1700 BASE PAIRS long.

There are several types of gene, depending upon their function and in addition genes are said to be dominant or recessive. A dominant characteristic is one that occurs whenever the gene is present while the effect of a recessive gene (for example, a disease) requires that the gene be on both members of the chromosome pair that is, it must be *homozygous*.

GENITAL the term describing anything relating to reproduction or the reproductive organs.

GENITALIA the male or female reproductive organs, often referring to the external parts only.

GENITO-URINARY TRACT (urogenital in U.S.) the genital and urinary organs and associated structures: kidneys, ureter, bladder, urethra and genitalia.

GERMAN MEASLES (*or* **RUBELLA**) a highly infectious viral disease occurring mainly in childhood, but which is mild in effect. Spread occurs through close contact with infected individuals and there is an incubation period of two to three weeks. The symptoms include headache, shivering and sore throat with a slight fever. There is some swelling of the neck and soon after the onset a rash of pink spots appears, initially on the face and/or neck, and subsequently spreading over the body. The rash disappears in roughly one week but the condition remains infectious for 3 or 4 more days.

Immunity is usually conferred by the infection and although it is a mild disease it is important because an attack during the early stages of pregnancy may cause foetal abnormalities. Girls are therefore immunized around the age of 12 or 13.

GERMS microorganisms. The term is used particularly for microorganisms that are PATHOGENIC.

GESTATION the length of time from fertilization of the ovum to birth (*see also* PREGNANCY).

GIDDINESS *see* VERTIGO.

GINGIVITIS inflammation of the gums.

GLAND an organ or group of cells that secretes a specific substance or substances. ENDOCRINE GLANDS secrete directly into the blood while *exocrine* glands secrete onto an epithelial surface via a duct. Some glands produce fluids, e.g. milk from the mammary glands, saliva from the sublingual bland and others. The THYROID gland is an endocrine gland releasing hormones into the bloodstream. A further system of glands, the lymphatic glands, occur throughout the body in association with the lymphatic vessels (*see* LYMPH).

GLANDULAR FEVER (*also known as* **INFECTIOUS MONO-NUCLEOSIS**) an infectious viral disease caused by the Epstein-Barr virus. It produces a sore throat and swelling in neck lymph nodes (also those in the armpits and groin). Other symptoms include headache, fever and a loss of appetite. The liver may be affected and the SPLEEN may become enlarged or even ruptured which then requires surgery. The disease is diagnosed by the large number of MONOCYTES in the blood and although complications tend to be rare, total recovery may take many weeks.

GLAUCOMA a condition which

results in loss of vision due to high pressure in the EYE, although there is usually no associated disease of the eye. There are several types of glaucoma which occur at differing rates but all are characterized by high intra-ocular pressure (due to the outflow of AQUEOUS HUMOUR being restricted) which damages nerve fibres in the RETINA and optic nerve. Treatment involves reduction of the pressure with drops and tablets (to reduce production of aqueous humour) and if necessary surgery is undertaken to create another outlet for the aqueous humour.

GLOTTIS the opening between the VOCAL CHORDS. Also used for the part of the LARYNX involved with sound production.

GLUCAGON a hormone important in maintaining the level of the body's blood sugar. It works antagonistically with INSULIN, increasing the supply of blood sugar through the breakdown of GLYCOGEN to glucose in the liver. Glucagon is produced by the ISLETS OF LANGER-HANS when blood sugar level is low.

GLUE EAR (*or* **SECRETORY OTITIS MEDIA**) a form of OTITIS, common in children, which occurs as an inflammation of the middle ear with the production of a persistent sticky fluid. It can cause deafness and may be associated with enlarged adenoids. In treatment of the condition the adenoids may be removed and grommets inserted.

GLUTEAL the term given to the buttocks or the muscles forming them.

GLUTEUS one of the three muscles of each buttock. The *gluteus maximus* shapes the buttock and extends the thigh, the *gluteus medius* and *minimus* abduct (move the limb away from the body) the thigh while the former also rotates it.

GOITRE swelling of the neck due to THYROID GLAND enlargement. The thyroid tries to counter the dietary lack of iodine necessary to produce thyroid hormone, by increasing the output, thereby becoming larger. The endemic or simple goitre is due to this cause. Other types are caused by HYPERPLASIA and auto-immune diseases, for example when antibodies are produced against antigens in the thyroid gland.

GONAD the reproductive organs that produce the GAMETES and some hormones. In the male and female the gonads are the testes and ovaries respectively.

GONADOTROPHIN (or GONADOTROPHIC HORMONE) hormones secreted by the anterior PITUITARY GLAND. Follicle-stimulating hormone (FSH) is produced by males and females as is luteinizing hormone, LH, (interstitial cell-stimulating hormone, ICSH, in males). FSH controls, directly or indirectly, growth of the ova and sperm, while LH/ICSH stimulates reproductive activity in the GONADS.

GOUT a disorder caused by an imbalance of uric acid in the body. Uric acid is normally excreted by the kidneys but sufferers of gout have an excess in their bloodstream which is deposited in joints as salts (urates) of the acid. This causes inflammation of the affected joints and painful gouty arthritis with destruction of the joints. The kidneys may also be damaged, with formation of stones. Deposits of the salts (called *tophi*) may reach the stage where they prohibit further use of the joints, causing hands and feet to be set in a particular position. Treatment of gout is through drugs that increase the excretion of the urate salts or slow their formation.

GRAAFIAN FOLLICLE *see* FOLLICLE.

GRAFT the removal of some tissue or an organ from one person for application to or implantation into the same person or another individual. For example, a skin graft involves taking healthy skin from one area of the body to heal damaged skin, and a kidney (or renal) graft (or transplant) is the removal of the organ from one person (usually a recently dead individual) to another. Numerous types of graft are now feasible, including skin, bone, cornea, cartilage, nerves and blood vessels, and whole organs such as kidney, heart and lung.

GRAM'S STAIN a technique described by H.C.J. Gram, the Danish bacteriologist in 1884, which involves using a stain to differentiate between certain bacteria. Bacteria on a microscope slide are first stained with a violet dye and iodine, then rinsed in ethanol to decolorize and a second red stain added. *Gram-positive* bacteria keep the first stain and appear violet when examined under the microscope, while *Gram-negative* forms lose the first but take up the second stain, thus appearing red. The difference in staining is due to the structure of the bacteria cell walls.

GRAND MAL a convulsive epileptic fit involving involuntary muscular contractions and lack of respiration. The latter produces bluish skin and lips (CYANOSIS) during the *tonic* phase. Convulsive movements follow and often the tongue is bitten and bladder control is lost (the *clonic* phase). Upon awakening the patient has no recall of the event.

GRANULOCYTE *see* LEUCOCYTE.

GRAVID another term for pregnant.

GREY MATTER a part of the CENTRAL NERVOUS SYSTEM comprising the central part of the spinal cord and the cerebral cortex and outer layer of the cerebellum in the brain. It is brown-grey in colour and is the co-ordination point between the nerves of the central nervous system.

It is composed of nerve cell bodies, DENDRITES, SYNAPSES, glial cells (supporting cells) and blood vessels.
GROIN the areas where the abdomen joins the thighs.
GROWTH HORMONE (somatotrophin or FH) a HORMONE produced and stored by the anterior PITUITARY GLAND that controls protein synthesis in muscles and the growth of long bones in legs and arms.

H

HAEMATEMESIS vomiting of blood which may occur for a number of different reasons. Common causes are ulcers, either gastric or duodenal, or gastritis, especially when this is caused by irritants or poisons such as alcohol.
HAEMATOCOELE leakage of blood into a cavity causing a swelling. A haematocoele usually forms as a result of an injury due to the rupture of blood vessels and the leaking of blood into a natural body cavity.
HAEMATOMA a collection of blood forming a firm swelling—a bruise. It may occur as a result of injury, a clotting disorder of the blood or if blood vessels are diseased.
HAEMATURIA the presence of blood in the urine which may have come from the kidneys, ureters, bladder or urethra. It indicates the presence of inflammation or disease such as a stone in the bladder or kidney.
HAEMOGLOBIN the respiratory substance contained within the red blood cells which contains a pigment responsible for the red colour of blood. It consists of the pigment HAEM and the protein globin and is responsible for the transport of

oxygen around the body. Oxygen is picked up in the lungs by arterial blood and transported to the tissues where it is released. This (venous) blood is then returned to the lungs to repeat the process, *see* OXYHAEMO-GLOBIN.
HAEMORRHAGE bleeding - a flow of blood from a ruptured blood vessel which may occur externally or internally. A haemorrhage is classified according to the type of vessels involved: *Arterial H* - bright red blood spurts in pulses from an artery. *Venous H* - a darker coloured steady flow from a vein. *Capillary L* - blood oozes from torn capillaries at the surface of a wound. In addition, a haemorrhage may be *primary* i.e. it occurs at the moment of injury. It is classed as *reactionary* when it occurs within 24 hours of an injury and results from a rise in blood pressure. Thirdly, a *secondary haemorrhage* occurs after a week or ten days as a result of infection (sepsis). Haemorrhage from a major artery is the most serious kind as large quantities of blood are quickly lost and death can occur within minutes.
HAEMORRHOIDS (piles) varicose and inflamed veins around the lower end of the bowel situated in the wall of the anus. They are classified as internal, external and mixed depending upon whether they appear beyond the anus. They are commonly caused by constipation or diarrhoea, especially in middle and older age, and may be exacerbated by a sedentary life style. They may also occur as a result of child-bearing.
HAEMOSTASIS the natural process to arrest bleeding involving blood coagulation and contraction of a ruptured blood vessel. The term is also applied to a number of surgical procedures designed to arrest bleeding such as the use of ligatures and diathermy. A haemostatic

substance stops or prevents haemorrhage e.g. phytomenadone.

HAEMOTHORAX a leakage of blood into the pleural cavity of the chest, usually as a result of injury.

HAMSTRING any of four tendons at the back of the knee which are attached to the *hamstring muscles* and anchor these to the TIBIA and FIBULA. The hamstring muscles are responsible for the bending of the knee joint.

HAND the extremity of the upper limb below the wrist which has a highly complex structure and an 'opposable' thumb which is unique to man. The human hand is highly developed in terms of structure, nervous supply and function and communicates with a large area on the surface of the brain. It is capable of performing numerous functions with a high degree of precision. When there is brain damage and paralysis, the uses of the hand tend to be lost early and more permanently compared to movements in the leg and face. The skeletal structure of the hand consists of eight small *carpal* bones in the wrist, five *metacarpal* bones in the region of the palm and three *phalanges* in each finger.

HAY FEVER an allergic reaction to pollen e.g. that of grasses, trees and many other plants which affects numerous individuals. The symptoms are a blocked and runny nose, sneezing and watering eyes due to the release of histamine. Treatment is by means of antihistamine drugs and, if the allergen can be identified, *desensitization* may be successful. This involves injecting or exposing the individual to controlled and gradually increasing doses of the allergen until antibodies are built up.

HEADACHE pain felt within the head which is thought to be caused by dilation of intracranial arteries or pressure upon them. Common causes

are stress, tiredness, feverishness accompanying an infection such as a cold, an excess of close work involving the eyes, dyspepsia, rheumatic diseases, high blood pressure and uraemia. Headache may indicate the presence of disease or disorder in the brain e.g. an infection such as MENINGITIS, TUMOUR or ANEURYSM and also as a result of injury and concussion.

HEART the hollow, muscular organ which acts as a pump and is responsible for the circulation of the blood. The heart is cone-shaped with the point downwards and is situated between the lungs and slightly to the left of the midline. The heart projects forwards and lies beneath the fifth rib. The wall consists mainly of CARDIAC MUSCLE lined on the inside by a membrane known as the ENDOCARDIUM. An external membrane known as the PERICARDIUM surrounds the heart. A SEPTUM divides the heart into right and left halves, each of which is further divided into an upper chamber known as an ATRIUM and a lower one called a VENTRICLE. Four valves control the direction of blood flow at each outlet, comprising the aortic, pulmonary, tricuspid and mitral (bicuspid). These valves prevent backflow once the blood has been forced from one chamber into the next. *See* CIRCULATION OF THE BLOOD.

HEART ATTACK *see* CARDIAC ARREST.

HEART BLOCK a condition describing a failure in the conduction of electrical impulses from the natural pacemaker (the sinoatrial node) through the heart, which can lead to slowing of the pumping action.

There are three types: in first degree (partial or incomplete) heart block there is a delay in conduction between atria (*see* ATRIUM) and VENTRICLES but this does not cause slowing. In second degree heart block, there is intermittent slowing because not all the impulses are conducted between atria and ventricles. In third degree (or complete) heart block there is no electrical conduction, the heartbeats are slow and the ventricles beat at their own intrinsic slow rhythm. This causes blackouts and can lead to heart failure.

HEARTBURN a burning pain or discomfort felt in the region of the heart and often rising upwards to the throat. It is caused by regurgitation of the stomach contents, the burning being caused by the acid in gastric juice or by oesophagitis. It is relieved by taking antacid tablets or alkaline substances such as sodium bicarbonate.

HEAT EXHAUSTION exhaustion and collapse due to overheating of the body and loss of fluid following unaccustomed or prolonged exposure to excessive heat. It is more common in hot climates and results from excessive sweating leading to loss of fluids and salts and disturbance of the electrolyte balance in body fluids. In the mildest form which is *heat collapse*, blood pressure and pulse rate fall accompanied by fatigue, light-headedness and there may be muscular cramps. Treatment involves taking drinks of salt solution, or these may be given intravenously and avoidance by gradual acclimatization to the heat, especially if hard physical work is to be carried out.

HEAT STROKE or **HEAT HYPER-PYREXIA** a severe condition following exposure of the body to excessive heat characterized by a rise in temperature and failure of sweating and temperature regulation. There is a loss of consciousness, followed by coma and death which can occur rapidly. The body must be cooled by

sponging and salt solutions given either by mouth or intravenously.

HEEL the part of the foot behind the ankle joint formed by the *calcaneus* or heel bone.

HEIMLICH'S MANOEUVRE a procedure to dislodge a foreign body which is blocking the larynx causing choking.

HEPATITIS inflammation of the liver due to the presence of toxic substances or infection caused by viruses. *Acute hepatitis* produces abdominal pain, jaundice, itching, nausea and fever. *Chronic hepatitis* has a similar range of symptoms which may persist for years and lead eventually to CIRRHOSIS. Alcohol abuse is a common cause of hepatitis which may also result as a side effect from a number of drug treatments or from overdose. Many virus infections can cause hepatitis such as HIV and GLANDULAR FEVER. However, the so-called hepatic viruses are designated A, B, C, D, and E. Hepatitis A causes *infectious hepatitis* (epidemic hepatitis) and is transmitted by eating food contaminated by a person who has the virus, and is common in conditions of poor hygiene and sanitation. Hepatitis E acts in a similar way and both produce symptoms of fever, sickness and jaundice. Recovery is usually complete unless the symptoms are acute and immunity from a future attack is conferred. *Serum hepatitis* is caused by viruses B, C and D, the route of infection being blood or blood products. Serum hepatitis is most common where infected needles have been used among drug addicts. The infection may also be passed on by tattooing needles and also through sexual intercourse with an infected individual. The mortality rate is 5 - 20%, but many patients make a gradual recovery from the illness which is characterized by fever, chills, fatigue, headaches and jaundice. All these viruses may persist in the blood for a long time and if B is involved, the condition is known as *chronic type - B hepatitis*.

HERNIA the protrusion of a part or whole of an organ from out of its normal position within the body cavity. Most commonly, a hernia involves part of the bowel. A *congenital hernia* is present at birth, a common one being an *umbilical hernia* in which abdominal organs protrude into the umbilical cord. This is due to a failure during foetal development and can be corrected by surgery. An *acquired hernia* occurs after birth, a common example being an *inguinal hernia* in which part of the bowel bulges through a weak part of the abdominal wall, (known as the inguinal canal). Another common type is a *hiatus hernia* in which the stomach passes through the hiatus (a hole allowing passage of the oesophagus), from the abdomen into the chest cavity. A *reducible hernia* is freely movable and can be returned by manipulation into its rightful place. An *irreducible hernia* describes the opposite situation and an *incarcerated hernia* is one which has become swollen and fixed in its position. An *obstructed hernia* is one involving the bowel. The contents of the hernia are unable to pass further down and are held up and obstructed.
The most dangerous situation is a *strangulated hernia* in which the blood supply has been cut off due to the protrusion itself. This becomes painful and eventually gangrenous and requires immediate surgery. Strenuous physical activity can lead to a hernia which usually develops gradually. Although short-term measures are employed to control a hernia or reduce its size, the usual treatment is by means of surgery to return and retain the protrusion in its proper pace.

HERPES infectious inflammation of the skin and mucous membranes, characterized by the development of small blisters, and caused by a number of different *Herpes viruses*. The *Herpes simplex* virus, types I and II, are the cause of cold sores which usually affect the lips, mouth and face. The virus is usually acquired in childhood and once present persists for life. It can be contracted without causing any symptoms but tends to flare up from time to time producing the cold sores.
Herpes simplex is also the cause of genital herpes in which the blisters affect the genital region. *Herpes zoster* or shingles is produced by a virus which causes chicken pox in children. The virus affects the course of a nerve producing severe pain and small yellowish blisters on the skin. Often the affected areas are the abdomen, back, face and chest and although the disease subsides after about three weeks, the blisters form scabs which eventually drop off and the pain can persist for months. This is known as *post-herpetic neuralgia* and pain-relieving drugs are needed to help relieve the condition.

HIATUS HERNIA *see* HERNIA.

HINDBRAIN the part of the brain which consists of the MEDULLA OBLONGATA, PONS and CEREBELLUM.

HIP the region on either side of the body where the FEMUR (thigh bone) articulates with the pelvis.

HISTAMINE a substance derived from histidine which is an amino acid. It is widely found throughout all the body tissues and is responsible for the dilation of blood vessels (arterioles and capillaries) and the contraction of smooth muscle, including that of the bronchi of the lungs. Histamine is released in great quantities in allergic conditions and ANAPHYLAXIS (*see also* ALLERGY).

HIV the *H*uman *I*mmunodeficiency *V*irus responsible for the condition known as AIDS. The virus affects and destroys a group of lymphocytes (T-lymphocytes) which are part of the body's natural defences (the IMMUNE SYSTEM).

HIVES a common name for urticaria or nettle rash.

HORMONE a naturally-produced chemical substance produced by the body which acts as a messenger. A hormone is produced by cells or glands in one part of the body and passes into the bloodstream. When it reaches another specific site, its 'target organ,' it causes a reaction there, modifying the structure or function of cells, perhaps by causing the release of another hormone. Hormones are secreted by the ENDOCRINE GLANDS and examples are the sex hormones, e.g. TESTOSTERONE secreted by the testes and oestradiol and PROGESTER-ONE secreted by the ovaries.

HUMERUS the bone of the upper arm which articulates with the shoulder blade (SCAPULA) of the PECTORAL GIRDLE and the ULNA and RADIUS at the elbow.

HUMOUR a natural fluid in the body, the best known examples being the aqueous and vitreous humours of the EYE.

HYDROCEPHALUS an abnormal collection of cerebrospinal fluid within the skull which causes, in babies and children, a great increase in the size of the head. Hydrocephalus results either from an excessive production of fluid or from a defect in the mechanism for its reabsorption, or from a blockage in its circulation. The cause may be CONGENITAL, and it often accompanies SPINA BIFIDA in babies, or infection (meningitis) or the presence of a TUMOUR. Hydrocephalus causes pressure on the brain with drowsiness, irritability and mental subnormality in children.

HYPERALGESIA an extreme sensitivity to pain.

HYPERGLYCAEMIA the presence of excess sugar (glucose) in the blood, as in DIABETES MELLITUS caused by insufficient INSULIN to cope with carbohydrate intake. The condition can lead to a diabetic coma.

HYPERPLASIA increased growth in size and number of the normal cells of a tissue so that the affected part enlarges e.g. the breasts during pregnancy. Compare HYPERTROPHY and NEOPLASM.

HYPERSENSITIVITY abnormal allergic response to an ANTIGEN to which the person has previously been exposed. Hypersensitive responses vary from quite mild such as hay fever to very severe and life-threatening e.g. ANAPHYLACTIC SHOCK (see also ALLERGY).

HYPERTENSION high blood pressure (in the arteries). Essential hypertension may be due to an unknown cause, or kidney disease or endocrine diseases. Malignant hypertension will prove fatal if not treated. It may be a condition itself or an end stage of essential hypertension. It tends to occur in a younger age group and there is high diastolic blood pressure (see DIASTOLE) and kidney failure. Previously a rapidly fatal condition, antihypertensive drugs have revolutionized treatment and given sufferers a near-normal life.

HYPERTHERMIA extremely high and abnormal body temperature i.e. a fever. Also, a method of treatment of certain diseases by artificially inducing a state of fever achieved by a variety of techniques.

HYPERTROPHY an increase in the size of an organ due to enlargement of its cells (rather than in their number) often in response to a greater demand for work. An example is the increase in size of the remaining kidney if the other is removed for some reason. Compare HYPERPLASIA.

HYPERVENTILATION breathing at an abnormally rapid rate when at rest, which may be a response to stress and, if not checked, results in unconsciousness because the concentration of carbon dioxide in the blood falls. If the carbon dioxide level in the blood is abnormally high, due to impaired gas exchange in the lungs, e.g. in pulmonary OEDEMA and pneumonia, hyperventilation may occur. (*See also* HYPOVENTILATION.)

HYPODERMIC beneath the skin. The term is usually used in reference to injections given by means of a *hypodermic syringe.*

HYPOGLYCAEMIA a lack of sugar in the blood which occurs in starvation and also with DIABETES MELLITUS when too much insulin has been given and insufficient carbohydrates have been eaten. The symptoms include weakness, sweating, light-headedness and tremors and can lead to coma. The symptoms are alleviated by taking in glucose either by mouth, or injection in the case of hypoglycæmic coma.

HYPOTHALAMUS an area of the forebrain in the floor of the third ventricle, having the thalamus above and pituitary gland below. It contains centres controlling vital processes, e.g. fat and carbohydrate metabolism, thirst and water regulation, hunger and eating, thermal regulation and sexual function. It also plays a part in the emotions and in the regulation of sleep. It controls the sympathetic and parasympathetic nervous systems and secretions from the pituitary gland.

HYPOTHERMIA describes the bodily state when the core temperature falls below 35°C due to prolonged exposure to cold. At first, shivering occurs and the heart works harder to increase the flow of blood around the body. However, eventually shivering ceases and, with increasing chilling, the function of the body organs becomes disturbed and cardiac output falls. The tissues require less oxygen as their functions start to fail, but eventually the heart is unable to supply even this reduced demand. The symptoms of hypothermia are fatigue and confusion followed by unconsciousness and death. The elderly are particularly at risk through inadequate domestic heating.

HYPOVENTILATION an abnormally slow rate of shallow breathing which may result from injury or the effects of drugs on the respiratory centre in the brain. The effect is to increase the amount of carbon dioxide in the blood and lessen that of oxygen. Eventually this leads to death due to a lack of oxygen supply to cells and tissues.

I

IDIOPATHIC the term given to a disease indicating that its cause is not known.

ILEITIS inflammation of the ILEUM with pain, bowel irregularity and loss of weight. The intestine may become thickened and if the tract becomes blocked, surgery is required immediately. The specific cause is not known but it may occur in association with tuberculosis, bacterial infection (by *Yersinia enterocolitica*), Crohn's disease (chronic inflammation of the bowel) and typhoid.

ILEUM the lower part of the small intestine between the JEJUNUM and the CAECUM.

ILEUS an obstruction of the intestine (often the ILEUM) which may be mechanical due to worms or a gallstone from the gall bladder, or it can be due to loss of the natural movement of the intestines (peristalsis). This latter condition may be caused by surgery, injury to the spine or PERITONITIS.

ILIAC ARTERIES those arteries supplying blood to the lower limbs and pelvic region.

ILIUM the largest of the bones that form each half of the pelvic girdle. It has a flattened wing-like part fastening to the SACRUM by means of ligaments.

IMMUNE the state of being protected against an infection by the presence of antibodies specific to the organism concerned.

IMMUNITY the way in which the body resists infection due to the presence of ANTIBODIES and white blood cells. Antibodies are generated in response to the presence of ANTIGENS of a disease. There are several types of immunity: *active immunity* is when the body produces antibodies and continues to be able to do so, during the course of a disease whether occurring naturally (also called *acquired immunity*) or by deliberate stimulation. *Passive immunity* is short-lived and due to the injection of ready-made antibodies from someone who is already immune.

IMMUNIZATION producing immunity to disease by artificial means. Injection of an antiserum will produce temporary passive immunity. Active immunity is produced by making the body generate its own antibodies and this is done by the use of treated antigens (vaccination or INOCULATION). VACCINE is used for immunization and it may be treated live bacteria or viruses or dead organisms or their products.

IMMUNOGLOBULINS a group of high molecular weight proteins that act as ANTIBODIES and are present in the SERUM and secretions. Designated Ig, there are five groups each with different functions identified by a particular letter.

IMPACTION a descriptive term for things being locked or wedged together; or stuck in position. For example a wisdom tooth is impacted when it cannot erupt normally because of other tissues blocking it.

IMPETIGO a staphylococcal and infectious skin disease found primarily in children. It spreads quickly over the body, starting as a red patch which forms pustules that join to create crusted yellowish sores. It is easily spread by contact or through towels etc. and must be treated quickly otherwise it may continue on an individual for months. Treatment with antibiotics is usually effective.

INCISION a surgical cut into tissue or organ, and the act of making the cut.

INCISOR the tooth with a chisel edge to it, used for biting. They form the four front teeth in each jaw.

INCONTINENCE an inability to control bowel movements or the passage of urine. Urinary incontinence may be due to a lesion in the brain or spinal cord, injury to the sphincter, or damage to the nerves of the bladder. Stress incontinence occurs during coughing or straining and is common in women due to weakening of muscles through childbirth.

INCUBATION 1. the time between a person being exposed to an infection and the appearance of symptoms. Incubation periods for diseases tend to be quite constant. 2. the time taken to start and grow microorganisms in culture media. 3. the process of caring for a premature baby in an incubator.

INDIGESTION *see* DYSPEPSIA.

INFARCTION the formation of an *infarct* or dead area of tissue in an organ or vessel due to the obstruction of the artery supplying blood. The obstruction may be caused by a blood clot or an EMBOLUS.

INFECTION when PATHOGENS invade the body causing disease. Bacteria, viruses, fungi etc. are all included and they enter the body, multiply and after the INCUBATION period symptoms appear. The organisms reach the body in many ways: airborne droplets, direct contact, sexual intercourse, by VECTORS, from contaminated food or drink etc.

INFERTILITY when a couple are unable to produce offspring naturally. Female infertility may be because of irregular or no ovulation, blocked FALLOPIAN TUBES, ENDOMETRI-OSIS; while a low sperm count or other deficiency in the spermatozoa can lead to male infertility. Treatment can include drug therapy, surgery, or more recently the technique of *in vitro* fertilization.

INFESTATION when animal parasites occur on the skin, in the hair or within the body (e.g. parasitic worms).

INFLAMMATION the response of the body's tissues to injury which involves pain, redness, heat and swelling (*acute* inflammation). The first sign when the tissues are infected or injured physically or chemically is a dilation of blood vessels in the affected area increasing blood flow resulting in heat and redness. The circulation then slows a little and white blood cells migrate into the tissues producing the swelling. The white blood cells engulf invading bacteria, dead tissue, foreign particles. After this either the white blood cells migrate back to the circulation, or there is the production and discharge of pus, as healing commences. *Chronic* inflammation is when repair is not complete and there is formation of scar tissue.

INFLUENZA a highly infectious disease caused by virus that affects the respiratory tract. Symptoms include headache, weakness and fever, appetite loss and general aches and pains. Sometimes there is the complication of a lung infection which requires immediate treatment. There are three main strains of influenza virus, designated A, B and C. The viruses quickly produce new strains which is why an attack of one is unlikely to provide protection against a later bout of the disease. Epidemics occur periodically and in Britain virus A is responsible for the majority of outbreaks.

INGESTION the process of chewing and swallowing food and fluid which then goes into the stomach. Also the means whereby a *phagocyte* (a cell that can surround and break down cell debris, foreign particles and microorganisms) takes in particles.

INHALANTS substances taken into the body by INHALATION. The substances can be in several forms: inhaling the steam of a hot solution; as a pressurized aerosol of droplets of particles; or as a non-pressurized passive inhaler where powdered medication is drawn into the body by inhaling deeply. Sufferers of asthma use inhalers to deliver drugs to the bronchi (bronchodilator drugs) for relief from attacks.

INHALATION 1. (*or* INSPIRA-TION) the act of drawing air into the lungs. 2. the medication breathed in, whether in gas, vapour of particulate form, to ensure contact with and/or treatment of conditions of the throat, bronchi or lungs.

INJECTION the means whereby a liquid (often a drug) is introduced into the body using a syringe when it would otherwise be destroyed by digestive processes. The location of the injection depends upon the speed with which the drug is to be absorbed and the target site. Thus injections may go into the skin (*intradermal*), beneath the skin

(*subcutaneous*, as with INSULIN). For
slow absorption an *intramuscular*
injection would be used, and
intravenous for fast delivery.

INNER EAR *see* EAR.

INOCULATION the process
whereby a small quantity of material
is introduced into the body to
produce or increase immunity to the
disease related to the injected
material (*see* IMMUNIZATION *and*
VACCINATION).

INSULIN a pancreatic hormone
produced in the ISLETS OF LANGERHANS
that initiates uptake of glucose by
body cells and thereby controls the
level of glucose in the blood. It
works by stimulating proteins on cell
surfaces within muscles and other
tissues to take up the glucose for
their activity. A lack of hormone
results in the sugar derived from
food being excreted in the urine - the
condition DIABETES MELLITUS. For such
cases, insulin can be administered by
injection.

INTERCOSTAL the term given to
nerves, muscles etc. that are situated
between the ribs.

INTERVERTEBRAL DISC fibrous
cartilaginous discs that connect
adjacent vertebrae and permit
rotational and bending movements.
The discs make up approximately
25% of the backbone length and they
act as shock absorbers providing
cushioning for the brain and spinal
cord. With age the discs lose their
effectiveness and may be displaced.

INTESTINE the part of the
ALIMENTARY CANAL or tract between
stomach and anus where final
digestion and absorption of food
matter occur in addition to the
absorption of water and production
of faeces. The intestine is divided
into the small intestine comprising
DUODENUM, ILEUM and JEJUNUM, and the
large intestine made up of the
CAECUM, vermiform APPENDIX, COLON
and RECTUM. The length of the

intestine in man is about 30 feet.

INTOXICATION being poisoned
by drugs, alcohol or other toxic
substances.

INTRACRANIAL term meaning
within the skull and applied to
diseases, structures etc.

INTRACRANIAL PRESSURE the
pressure within the cranium, more
specifically the pressure as
maintained by all tissues: brain,
blood, cerebrospinal fluid etc. An
increase in the pressure can occur
through injury, haemorrhage, tumour
and treatment will be necessary.

INTRAMUSCULAR term meaning
within a muscle, as with an
intramuscular injection.

INTRAVENOUS term meaning
relating to the inside of a vein hence
intravenous injections are made into
a vein, and blood transfusions are
intravenous.

INTUBATION the insertion of a
tube into the body through a natural
opening. It is commonly, though not
exclusively, used to keep an airway
open by insertion into the mouth or
nose into the larynx. The same
technique may be adopted to enable
an anaesthetic gas, or oxygen to be
delivered.

INVASION when bacteria enter the
body; but more commonly used to
describe the process whereby
malignant cancer cells move into
nearby normal and deeper tissues
and gain access to the blood vessels.

IRIS the part of the EYE that controls
the amount of light to enter. It is in
effect a muscular disc and to reduce
the amount of light entering circular
muscles contract, and to increase the
aperture in dim light, radiating
muscles contract. The varying sized
hole is the PUPIL. The iris can be seen
through the CORNEA which is
transparent and is the coloured part
of the eye, this latter feature is due to
pigment cells containing melanin
(blue is little; brown is more).

IRRIGATION the washing out of a wound or body cavity with a flow of water or other fluid.

IRRITANT a general term encompassing any agent that causes irritation of a tissue e.g. nettle stings, chemicals and gases etc.

ISCHAEMIC relating to a decrease in blood supply to a part of the body or an organ, caused by a blockage or narrowing of the blood vessels. It is often associated with pain.

ISCHIUM one of the three bones that comprise each half of the pelvis. It is the most posterior and it supports the weight of the body when sitting.

ISLETS OF LANGERHANS clusters of cells within the PANCREAS which are the ENDOCRINE part of the gland. There are three types of cells termed alpha, beta and delta, the first two producing GLUCAGON and INSULIN respectively, both vital hormones in the regulation of blood sugar levels. The third hormone produced is somatostatin (also released by the HYPOTHALAMUS) which works antagonistically against growth hormone by blocking its release by the pituitary gland. The islets were named after Paul Langerhans, a German pathologist.

ITCHING a skin condition or sensation prompting scratching to obtain relief. The causes are numerous and include mechanical irritation e.g. by clothing or lice, skin diseases or conditions such as ECZEMA, allergies etc.

J

JAUNDICE a condition character-ized by the unusual presence of bile pigment (BILIRUBIN) in the blood. The BILE produced in the liver passes into the blood instead of the intestines and because of this there is a yellowing of the skin and the whites of the eyes.

There are several types of jaundice: *obstructive* due to bile not reaching the intestine due to an obstruction e.g. a GALLSTONE; *haemolytic* where red blood cells are destroyed by HAEMOLYSIS; *hepatocellular* due to a liver disease such as HEPATITIS which results in the liver being unable to use the bilirubin. *Neonatal jaundice* is quite common in newborn infants when the liver is physio-logically immature but it usually lasts only a few days. The infant can be exposed to blue light which converts bilirubin to biliverdin, another (harmless) bile pigment.

JAW a term for the bones that carry the teeth and associated soft tissues. More specifically, they are the upper jaw (*maxilla*) and the lower jaw (*mandible*). The maxillae are fixed, while the mandible (which is one bone after the age of about 12 months) hinges on part of the temporal bone, in front of the ear.

JEJUNUM the part of the small intestine lying before the ILEUM and after the DUODENUM. Its main function is the absorption of digested food and its lining has numerous finger-like projections (villi) that increase the surface area for absor-ption. The villi are longer in the jejunum than elsewhere in the small intestine.

JOINTS connections between bones (and cartilages). Joints can be divided upon their structure and the degree to which they permit movement. *Fibrous* joints are fixed by fibrous tissue binding bones together e.g the bones of the skull. *Cartilaginous* joints are slightly movable. These have discs of cartilage between bones so that only limited movement is permitted over one joint but over several adjacent joints, considerable flexure is achieved, as with the spine. The final category is *synovial* joints which can move freely. Each synovial joint comprises the bones, cartilage over the ends, then a *capsule* (sheath of fibrous tissue) from which the ligaments form, and a SYNOVIAL MEMBRANE with synovial fluid to lubricate the joint.

This type of joint then occurs in two forms: hinge joints allowing planar movement (e.g. the knee) and ball and socket joints permitting all-round movement (e.g. the hip). Joints are subject to various conditions and diseases including SYNOVITIS, epiphysitis (inflammation of the EPIPHYSIS), GOUT, RHEUMATISM and dislocations.

JUGULAR a general term for structures in the neck.

JUGULAR VEIN any of the veins in the neck, particularly the anterior, internal and external. The anterior jugular vein is an offshoot of the external jugular and runs down the front of the neck. The external jugular itself drains the scalp, face and neck while the larger internal jugular drains the face, neck and brain and is sited vertically down the side of the neck.

K

KERNIG'S SIGN the inability of someone with MENINGITIS to straighten his legs at the knee when the thighs are at right angles to be body. It is symptomatic of the disease.

KETONE an organic compound that contains a carbonyl group (C=O) within the compound. Ketones can be detected in the body when fat is metabolized for energy when food intake is insufficient.

KIDNEY one of two glands/organs that remove nitrogenous wastes, mainly UREA, from the blood and also adjust the concentrations of various

salts. The kidney measures roughly 10cm long, 6cm wide and 4cm thick, and is positioned at the back of the abdomen, below the diaphragm. Blood is supplied to the kidney by the renal artery and leaves via the renal vein. Each kidney is held in place by fat and connective tissue and comprises an inner medulla and outer cortex. The kidneys produce and eliminate URINE by a complex process of filtration and reabsorption. The 'active' parts are the nephrons which filter blood under pressure, reabsorbing water and other substances. A nephron comprises a renal tubule and blood vessels. The tubule expands into a cup shape (*Bowman's capsule*) that contains a knot of capillaries (the *glomerulus*) and the latter bring the water, urea, salts, etc. Filtrate passes from the glomerulus through three areas of the tubule (proximal convoluted tubule; the loop of Henle, distal convoluted tube, which together form a shape resembling a hairpin) leaving as urine.

KNEE the joint connecting the thigh to the lower leg and formed by the femur, tibia and kneecap (PATELLA). It is a hinge type of synovial JOINT with very strong ligaments binding the bones together. Although the knee is a strong joint, it is complex and injuries can be serious.

KNEE JERK *see* REFLEX ACTION.

L

LABOUR the process of giving birth from dilatation of the CERVIX to expulsion of the afterbirth. It usually commences naturally although some labours are induced (*see* INDUCTION). The cervix expands and at the same time the muscles of the uterus wall contract pushing part of the AMNION down into the opening. The amnion ruptures releasing the 'waters' but these two events do not necessarily occur at the same time. The second stage is the actual delivery of the child which passes through the bony girdle of the pelvis, via the VAGINA to the outside. Initially the head appears at the cervix and the uterine contractions strengthen. These contractions are augmented by abdominal muscular contractions when the baby is in the vagina. When the baby's head is clear, the whole body is helped out and the umbilical cord severed. The final stage, accomplished by some contractions is expulsion of the PLACENTA and membranes.

On average, labour lasts 12 hours (less for subsequent pregnancies) and in the second stage an EPISIOTOMY may be necessary to facilitate the emergence of the head. In most cases, the baby lies head down at delivery although some are delivered feet or buttocks first (BREECH PRESENTATION). Other complications tend to be rare and maternal mortality is very low in the west.

LABYRINTH part of the inner ear (*see* EAR) consisting of canals, ducts and cavities forming the organs of hearing and balance. There are two parts; the *membranous labyrinth* comprising the semi-circular canals and associated structures and the central cavity of the cochlea, and the *bony labyrinth*, a system of canals filled with perilymph and surrounding the other parts.

LACERATION a wound with jagged edges.

LACRIMAL relating to, or about tears.

LACUNA (*plural* **LACUNAE**) an anatomical term meaning a small depression, cavity or pit, especially in compact bone.

LARGE INTESTINE *see* INTESTINE.

LARYNGITIS inflammation of the mucous membrane that lines the LARYNX and vocal cords. It is due to viral infection in the main, but also bacteria, chemical irritants, heavy smoking or excessive use of the voice. *Acute* laryngitis accompanies infections of the upper respiratory tract and the symptoms include pain, a cough, difficulty in swallowing. *Chronic* laryngitis may be due to recurrence of the acute form, but is often attributable to excessive smoking worsened by alcohol. Changes occurring in the vocal cords are more permanent and the symptoms are as for the acute form, but longer lasting.

LARYNGOTRACHEOBRON-CHITIS an acute inflammation of the major parts of the respiratory tract, causing shortness of breath, a croup-like cough and hoarseness. It occurs usually through viral infection and particularly in young children where there may be some obstruction of the LARYNX (*see also* CROUP). The main airways, bronchi, become coated with fluid generated by the inflamed tissues resulting in the shortness of breath. Treatment is through inhalations, antibiotics if appropriate and if the obstruction is serious, hospitalization may be necessary for INTUBATION, TRACHEOS-TOMY etc.

LARYNX part of the air passage connecting the PHARYNX with the TRACHEA and also the organ producing vocal sounds. It is situated high up in the front of the neck and is constructed of cartilages with ligaments and muscles. The ligaments bind together the cartilages and one pair of these form the VOCAL CORDS. The larynx is lined with mucous membrane and in all is about 5 cm long.

LAXATIVE a substance that is taken to evacuate the bowel or to soften stools. Typical laxatives include castor oil, senna, and its derivatives (*see also* PURGATIVE).

LEGIONNAIRE'S DISEASE a bacterial infection and a form of pneumonia caused by *Legionella pneumophila*. It produces an illness similar to influenza with symptoms appearing after a two to ten day incubation period. Fever, chills, head and muscular aches may progress to PLEURISY and chest pains. Antibiotic treatment is usually effective (e.g. erythromycin).

The bacterium is found in nature, particularly in water, and static water provides ideal conditions for multiplication. Inhalation of an aerosol of water is the likeliest way of becoming infected and air conditioning cooling towers are a particular source of infected water. It is vital that infected systems be cleaned and chlorinated.

LENS the part of the eye that focuses incoming light onto the RETINA. It is composed of a fibrous protein, crystallin, and is enclosed in a thin capsule.

LESION a wound or injury to body tissues. Also an area of tissue which because of damage due to disease or wounding does not function fully. Thus primary lesions include tumours and ulcers, and from primary lesions secondaries may form.

LETHARGY the state of being inactive mentally and physically and one that approaches the unconscious. The cause may be psychological or physical. The lethargy associated with the aftermath of glandular fever is well-known but it may also be due to ANAEMIA, DIABETES MELLITUS or malnutrition, amongst others.

LEUCOCYTE (or leukocyte) a white blood cell, so called because it contains no HAEMOGLOBIN. It also differs from red blood cells in having a nucleus. Leucocytes are formed in the bone marrow, spleen,

thymus and lymph nodes and there are three types: granulocytes, comprising 70% of all white blood cells, lymphocytes (25%) and monocytes (5%). Granulocytes help combat bacterial and viral infection and may be involved in allergies. LYM-PHOCYTES destroy foreign bodies either directly or through production of antibodies and MONOCYTES ingest bacteria and foreign bodies by the process called *phagocytosis* (engulfing micro-organisms and cell debris to remove them from the body). In disease, immature forms of leucocytes may appear in the blood (ultimately forming both red and white blood cells).

LEUKAEMIA a cancerous disease in which there is an uncontrolled proliferation of LEUCOCYTES in the bone marrow. The cells fail to mature to adult cells and thus cannot function as part of the defence mechanism against infections. This leads to anaemia, bleeding, easy bruising, with enlargement of the spleen, liver and lymph nodes. Acute leukaemia has a sudden onset and development while the chronic form may take years to develop the same symptoms.

LIGAMENT bands of fibrous connective tissue composed chiefly of COLLAGEN, that join bones together, restricting movement and preventing dislocation. Ligaments strengthen joints and most joints are surrounded by a capsular ligament. Also, a layer of SEROUS MEMBRANE e.g. the PERITONEUM that supports or links organs.

LIGATURE material for tying firmly around a blood vessel or duct to stop bleeding or prevent flow. The material may be wire, silk, catgut etc.

LIGHT REFLEX the mechanism whereby the PUPIL of the EYE opens in response to direct light or consensual pupillary stimulation (i.e. stimulation of one pupil with light results in a response from the other pupil).

LINGUAL term meaning relating to the tongue, or something close to the tongue e.g. lingual nerve, or the lingual surface of a tooth.

LINT a cotton fabric (formerly linen) used for surgical dressings which has one fluffy side and one smooth, the latter being placed against the skin.

LISTERIOSIS an infectious disease caused when the Gram-positive (*see* GRAM'S STAIN) bacterium *Listeria monocytogenes* which attacks animals is contracted by man through eating infected products. It produces symptoms similar to influenza or it may cause MENINGITIS or ENCEPHALITIS. The old and frail are more susceptible as are the new-born. It may terminate a pregnancy or damage the foetus if contracted during a pregnancy. Antibiotics such as penicillin provide an effective treatment.

LIVER a very important organ of the body, with many functions critical in regulating metabolic processes. It is also the largest gland in the body weighing around 1 kg. It occupies the top right hand part of the abdominal cavity and is made up of four lobes. It is fastened to the abdominal wall by ligaments and sits beneath the DIAPHRAGM, and upon the right kidney, large intestine, DUODENUM and stomach.

There are two blood vessels supplying the liver: the hepatic artery delivers oxygenated blood, while the hepatic portal vein conveys digested food from the stomach. Among its functions, the liver converts excess glucose to glycogen for storage as a food reserve; excess amounts of amino acids are converted to urea for excretion by the kidneys; BILE is produced for storage in the GALL BLADDER and lipolysis occurs; some poisons are broken down (detoxi-

fied) hence the beneficial effect of the hepatic portal vein carrying blood to the liver rather than it going around the body first.

The liver also synthesizes blood-clotting substances such as fibrinogen and prothrombin and the anti-coagulant heparin; it breaks down red blood cells at the end of their life and processes the haemoglobin for iron, which is stored; vitamin A is synthesized and stored and it also stores vitamins B_{12}, D, E and K. In the embryo it forms red blood cells. Such is the chemical and biochemical activity of the liver that significant heat energy is generated and this organ is a major contributor of heat to the body.

LOBE certain organs are divided by fissures into large divisions which are called lobes, e.g. the brain, liver and lungs.

LOCKJAW see TETANUS.

LOIN that area of the back between the lower ribs and pelvis.

LUMBAGO pain of any sort in the lower back. It can be muscular, skeletal or neurological in origin. A severe and sudden case may be due to a strained muscle or slipped disc and the latter is usually the cause of lumbago with SCIATICA.

LUMBAR a general term for anything relating to the LOINS, e.g. LUMBAR VERTEBRAE.

LUMBAR VERTEBRAE numbering five, the lumbar vertebrae are between the SACRUM and the thoracic vertebrae at the lowest part of the back. These vertebrae are not fused and have strong attachments points (processes) for the muscles of the lower back.

LUNGS the sac-like, paired organs of respiration situated with their base on the DIAPHRAGM and the top projecting into the neck. Each lung consists of fibrous, elastic sacs that are convoluted to provide a large surface area for gaseous exchange. Air enters the body through the windpipe or TRACHEA which branches into two bronchi (*see* BRONCHUS), one to each lung. Further branching then occurs, into numerous BRONCHIOLES. The bronchioles divide further and then end in alveoli (*see* ALVEOLUS) which are tiny sac-like structures where the gaseous exchange occurs. The exchange of oxygen and carbon dioxide occurs between the many blood capillaries on one side of the membrane and the air on the other. The lungs are served by the pulmonary arteries and pulmonary veins.

The *total lung capacity* of an adult male is five to six litres although only about half a litre (500ml) is exchanged in normal breathing (called the *tidal volume*).

LYMPH a colourless, watery fluid that surrounds the body tissues and circulates in the lymphatic system. It is derived from blood and is similar to plasma comprising 95% water, with protein, sugar, salts and lymphocytes. The lymph is circulated by muscular action and it passes through lymph nodes which act as filters, and is eventually returned to the blood via the thoracic duct (one of the two main vessels of the lymphatic system).

LYMPHATIC GLAND *see* GLAND.

LYMPHATICS (*or* **LYMPHATIC SYSTEM**) the network of vessels, valves, nodes etc. that carry lymph from the tissues to the bloodstream and help maintain the internal fluid environment of the body. Lymph drains into capillaries and larger vessels, passing through nodes and going eventually into two large vessels (the thoracic duct and right lymphatic duct) which return it to the bloodstream by means of the innominate veins.

LYSIS the destruction of cells by antibodies called *lysins*, thus haemolysis is the break-up of red blood cells by haemolysin. Also, more generally, the destruction of cells or tissues due to breakdown of the cell membranes.

M

MACULES spots of small pigmented areas in the skin which may be thickened. They appear as a result of pregnancy, sunburn, eczema, psoriasis and may be symptomatic of other diseases such as syphilis and those affecting internal organs.

MALABSORPTION SYNDROME a group of diseases in which there is a reduction in the normal absorption of digested food materials in the small intestine. The food materials involved are commonly fats, vitamins, minerals, amino acids and iron.

MALIGNANT a term used in several ways but commonly referring to a tumour that proliferates rapidly and destroys surrounding healthy tissue, and which can spread via the lymphatic and blood system to other parts of the body. The term is also applied to a more serious form of a disease than the usual one which is life-threatening such as *malignant smallpox* and malignant HYPERTENSION.

MAMMARY GLAND a gland present in the female breast which produces milk after childbirth.

MASTALGIA pain in the breast.

MASTOID PROCESS a projection of the temporal bone of the skull which contains numerous air spaces (mastoid cells) and is situated behind the ear. It provides a point of attachment for some of the neck muscles and communicates with the middle ear through an air-filled channel called the *mastoid antrum*.

MEASLES an extremely infectious

disease of children caused by a virus and characterized by the presence of a rash. It occurs in epidemics every two or three years. After an incubation period of 10 to 15 days the initial symptoms are those of a cold with coughing, sneezing and high fever. It is at this stage that the disease is most infectious and spreads from one child to another in airborne droplets before measles has been diagnosed. This is the main factor responsible for the epidemic nature of the disease. Small red spots with a white centre (known as *Koplik spots*) may appear in the mouth on the inside of the cheeks. Then a characteristic rash develops on the skin, spreading from behind the ears and across the face and also affecting other areas. The small red spots may be grouped together in patches and the child's fever is usually at its height while these are developing. The spots and fever gradually decline and no marks are left upon the skin, most children making a good recovery. However, complications can occur, particularly pneumonia and middle ear infections, which can result in deafness. A vaccine now available has reduced the incidence and severity of measles in the United Kingdom.

MEDIA the middle layer of a tissue or organ. Usually it is applied to the middle layer of the wall of a vein or artery comprising alternating sheaths of smooth muscle and elastic fibres.

MEDIASTINUM the space in the chest cavity between the two lungs which contains the heart, aorta, oesophagus, trachea, thymus gland and phrenic nerves.

MEDICATION any substance introduced into or on the body for the purposes of medical treatment, e.g. drugs and medicated dressings.

MEDULLA refers to the inner portion of a tissue or organ when there are two distinct parts. Examples include the adrenal medulla and the medulla of the kidneys. *Compare* CORTEX.

MEDULLA OBLONGATA the lowest part of the brain stem which extends through the FORAMEN *magnum* to become the upper part of the spinal cord. It contains important centres which govern respiration, circulation, swallowing and salivation.

MEGALOBLAST an abnormally large form of any of the cells that go on to produce erythrocytes (red blood cells). In certain forms of anaemia (megaloblastic anaemias) they are found in the bone marrow and their presence is due to a deficiency of vitamin B_{12} or of folic acid. They indicate a failure in the maturation process of erythrocytes which results in anaemia.

MELANIN a dark brown pigment found in the skin and hair and also in the choroid layer of the eye. Melanin is contained and produced within cells known as *melanocytes* in the dermis layer of the skin. When the skin is exposed to hot sunshine, more melanin is produced giving a 'suntan.' In dark-skinned races more melanin is produced by greater activity of the melanocytes and it helps to protect the skin from harmful ultra violet radiation.

MELANOMA an extremely malignant tumour of the melano-cytes, the cells in the skin which produce melanin. Melanomas are also found, although less commonly, in the mucous membranes and in the eye. There is a link between the occurrence of melanoma of the skin and exposure to harmful ultra violet light during sunbathing. A highly malignant form can also arise from the pigmented cells of moles. Melanoma can be successfully treated by surgery if it is superficial and caught at an early stage.

However, it commonly spreads, especially to the liver and lymph nodes, in which case the outlook is poor. The incidence of malignant melanoma is increasing and has attracted much attention in connection with the formation of holes in the ozone layer, which screens the earth from harmful UV radiation. Most experts recommend that people should cover exposed skin, use sunscreen creams and avoid the sun at the hottest part of the day.

MEMBRANE a thin composite layer of lipoprotein surrounding an individual cell or a thin layer of tissue surrounding an organ, lining a cavity or tube or separating tissues and organs within the body.

MENINGES the three connective tissue membranes which surround the spinal cord and brain. The outermost layer (meninx) is called the *dura mater* which is fibrous, tough and inelastic, and also called the *pachymeninx*, closely lining the inside of the skull and helping to protect the brain. It is thicker than the middle layer, the *arachnoid mater*, which surrounds the brain. The innermost layer, the *pia mater*, is thin and delicate and lines the brain. Cerebrospinal fluid circulates between it and the arachnoid mater and both these inner layers are richly supplied with blood vessels which supply the surface of the brain and skull. These two inner membranes are sometimes collectively called the *pia-arachnoid* or *leptomeninges*.

MENINGITIS inflammation of the meninges (membranes) of the brain (*cerebral meningitis*) or spinal cord (*spinal meningitis*) or the disease may affect both regions. Meningitis may affect the *dura mater* membrane in which case it is known as *pachymeningitis*, although this is relatively uncommon. It often results as a secondary infection due to the presence of disease elsewhere, as in

the case of *tuberculous meningitis* and *syphilitic meningitis*. Meningitis which affects the other two membranes, (the *pia-arachnoid* membranes) is known as *leptomeningitis* and this is more common and may be either a primary or secondary infection. Meningitis is also classified according to its causal organism and may be either viral or bacterial. *Viral meningitis* is fairly mild and as it does not respond to drugs, treatment is by means of bed rest until recovery takes place. *Bacterial meningitis* is much more common and is caused by the organisms responsible for tuberculosis, pneumonia and syphilis. Also, the *meningococcus* type of bacteria causes one of the commonest forms of the disease, *meningococcal meningitis*. The symptoms are a severe headache, sensitivity to light and sound, muscle rigidity especially affecting the neck, KERNIG'S SIGN, vomiting, paralysis, coma and death. These are caused by inflammation of the meninges and by a rise in INTRACRANIAL PRESSURE.

MESENTERY a double layer of the peritoneal membrane (PERITONEUM) which is attached to the back wall of the abdomen. It supports a number of abdominal organs including the stomach, small intestine, spleen and pancreas and contains associated nerves, lymph and blood vessels.

METABOLISM the sum of all the physical and chemical changes within cells and tissues that maintain life and growth. The breakdown processes which occur are known as *catabolic* (*catabolism*), and those which build materials up are called *anabolic* (*anabolism*). The term may also be applied to describe one particular set of changes e.g. *protein metabolism*. Basal metabolism is the minimum amount of energy required to maintain the body's vital processes e.g. heartbeat and respiration and is usually assessed by means of various measurements taken while a person is at rest.

METACARPAL BONE one of the five bones of the middle of the hand between the phalanges of the fingers and the CARPAL bones of the wrist forming the *metacarpus*. The heads of the metacarpal bones form the knuckles, *see* HAND.

METASTASIS the process by which a malignant tumour spreads to a distant part of the body, and also refers to the secondary growth that results from this. The spread is accomplished by means of three routes, the blood circulation, lymphatic system and across body cavities.

METATARSAL BONE one of the five bones in the foot lying between the toes and the TARSAL bones of the ankle, together forming the *metatarsus*. The metatarsal bones are equivalent to the METACARPAL BONES in the hand.

MICTURITION the act of urination.

MIDDLE EAR *see* EAR.

MIGRAINE a very severe throbbing headache, usually on one side of the head, which is often accompanied by disturbances in vision, nausea and vomiting. Migraine is a common condition and seems to be triggered by any one or several of a number of factors. These include anxiety, fatigue, watching television or video screens, loud noises, flickering lights (e.g. strobe lights) and certain foods such as cheese and chocolate or alcoholic drinks. The cause is unknown but thought to involve constriction followed by dilation of blood vessels in the brain and an outpouring of fluid into surrounding tissues. The attack can last up to 24 hours and treatment is by means of bed rest in a darkened, quiet room and pain-relieving drugs.

MISCARRIAGE *see* ABORTION.

MITOSIS the type of cell division undergone by most body cells by means of which growth and repair of tissues can take place. Mitosis involves the division of a single cell to produce two genetically identical daughter cells each with the full number of chromosomes, *compare* MEIOSIS.

MITRAL VALVE formerly known as the *bicuspid valve*, this is located between the atrium and ventricle of the left side of the heart attached to the walls at the opening between the two. It has two cusps or flaps and normally allows blood to pass into the ventricle from the atrium, but prevents any back flow.

MOLE a dark-coloured pigmented spot in the skin which is usually brown. It may be flat or raised and may have hair protruding from it. Some types can become malignant, *see* MELANOMA.

MONONUCLEOSIS *see* **GLANDULAR FEVER**.

MORBIDITY the state of being diseased, the *morbidity rate* being expressed as the number of cases of a disease occurring within a particular number of the population.

MORIBUND dying.

MORNING SICKNESS vomiting and nausea, most common during the first three months of pregnancy.

MOTOR NERVE a nerve containing motor neurone fibres which carries electrical impulses outwards from the central nervous system to a muscle or gland to bring about a response there.

MOTOR NEURONE one of the units or fibres of a MOTOR NERVE. An *upper motor neurone* is contained entirely within the central nervous system having its cell body in the brain and its *axon* (a long process) extending into the spinal cord where it SYNAPSES with other neurones. A *lower motor neurone* has its cell body in the spinal cord or brain stem and an axon that runs outwards via a spinal or cranial MOTOR NERVE to an effector muscle or gland, *see* NERVE.

MOUTH the opening which forms the beginning of the alimentary canal and in which food enters the digestive process. The entrance is guarded by the lips behind which lie the upper and lower sets of teeth embedded in the jaw. The roof of the mouth is called the palate, the front part being hard and immobile while behind lies the mobile soft palate. The tongue is situated behind the lower teeth and SALIVARY GLANDS which are present secrete saliva into the mouth through small ducts. Saliva contains the enzyme ptyalin which begins the breakdown of starch while the chewing action of the teeth and manipulation with the tongue reduces the food to a more manageable size so that it can be swallowed.

MUCOSA another term for MUCOUS MEMBRANE.

MUCOUS MEMBRANE a moist membrane which lines many tubes and cavities within the body and is lubricated with MUCUS. The structure of a mucous membrane varies according to its site and they are found, for example, lining the mouth, respiratory, urinary and digestive tracts. Each has a surface EPITHELIUM, a layer containing various cells and glands which secrete mucus. Beneath this lie connective tissue and muscle layers, the *laminae propria* and *muscularis mucosa* respectively, the whole forming a pliable layer.

MUCUS a slimy substance secreted by MUCOUS MEMBRANES as a lubricant, and composed mainly of glycoproteins of which the chief one is *mucin*. It is a clear viscous fluid which may contain enzymes and has a protective function. It is normally present in small amounts but the quantity increases if inflammation and/or infection is present.

MUMPS an infectious disease of childhood usually occurring in those between the ages of 5 to 15, and caused by a virus which produces inflammation of the *parotid salivary glands*. The incubation period is two to three weeks followed by symptoms including feverishness, headache, sore throat and vomiting, before or along with a swelling of the parotid gland on one side of the face. The swelling may be confined to one side or spread to the other side of the face and also may go on to include the *submaxillary* and *sublingual salivary glands* beneath the jaw. Generally after a few days the swelling subsides and the child recovers but remains infectious until the glands have returned to normal. The infection may spread to the pancreas and, in 15 to 30% of males, to the testicles. In adult men this can cause sterility. More rarely, inflammation in females can affect the ovaries and breasts, and MENINGITIS is another occasional complication, especially in adults. A protective vaccine is now available.

MUSCLE the contractile tissue of the body which produces movements of various structures both internally and externally. There are three types of muscle: 1. *striated* or *voluntary muscle* which has a striped appearance when viewed under a microscope and is attached to the skeleton. It is called 'voluntary' because it is under the control of the will and produces movements, for example, in the limbs. 2. *smooth* or *involuntary muscle* which has a plain appearance when viewed microscopically and is not under conscious control but is supplied by the autonomic nervous system. Examples are the muscles which supply the digestive and respiratory tracts. 3. *cardiac muscle*, the specialized muscle of the walls of the heart which is composed of a network of branching, elongated fibres which rejoin and interlock, each having a nucleus. It has a somewhat striated appearance and where there are junctions between fibres, irregular transverse bands occur known as *intercalated discs*. This muscle is involuntary and contracts and expands rhythmically throughout a person's life. However, rate of heart beat is affected by activity within the vagus nerve.

MUSCLE CRAMP *see* CRAMP.

MYALGIA pain in a muscle.

MYCOSIS any disease caused by fungi, e.g. thrush and ringworm.

MYELIN a sheath of phospholipid and protein that surrounds the axons of some NEURONS. It is formed by specialized cells known as *Schwann cells*, each of which encloses the axon in concentric folds of its cell membrane. These folds then condense to form myelin, the neuron then being described as *myelinated*. Schwann cells produce myelin at regular intervals along the length of the axon and electrical impulses pass more rapidly along myelinated nerve fibres than along non-myelinated ones.

MYELOID means like or relating to bone marrow or, like a *myelocyte*. This is a cell which is an immature type of granulocyte responsible for the production of white blood cells.

MYELOMA a malignant disease of the bone marrow in which tumours are present in more than one bone at the same time. The bones may show 'holes' when X-rayed due to typical deposits, and certain abnormal proteins may be present in the blood and urine. Treatment is by chemotherapy and radiotherapy. *Myelomatosis* is the production of myeloma which is usually fatal.

MYOCARDIAL INFARCTION *see* CORONARY THROMBOSIS.

MYOCARDITIS inflammation of the muscle in the wall of the heart.

MYOCARDIUM the middle of the three layers of the HEART wall which is the thick, muscular area. The outer layer is the *epicardium* (forming part of the *pericardium*) and the inner the *endocardium*.

MYOMETRIUM the muscular tissue of the WOMB, composed of smooth muscle and surrounding the ENDOMETRIUM. Its contractions are influenced by the presence of certain hormones and are especially strong during LABOUR.

MYOPIA short-sightedness corrected by wearing spectacles with concave lenses.

MYXOEDEMA a disease caused by under-activity of the thyroid gland (HYPOTHYROIDISM). There is a characteristic development of a dry, coarse skin and swelling of subcutaneous tissue. There is intellectual impairment with slow speech and mental dullness, lethargy, muscle pain, weight gain and constipation. The hair thins and there may be increased sensitivity to cold. As the symptoms are caused by the deficiency of thyroid hormones, treatment consists of giving THYROXINE in suitable amounts.

N

NARCOTIC a drug that leads to a stupor and complete loss of awareness. In particular opiates derived from morphine or produced synthetically produce various conditions: deep sleep, euphoria, mood changes and mental confusion. In addition, respiration and the cough reflex are depressed and muscle spasms may be produced.

NASAL CAVITY one of two cavities in the nose, divided by a SEPTUM, which lie between the roof of the mouth and the floor of the cranium.

NAUSEA a feeling of being about to vomit. It may be due to motion sickness, early pregnancy, pain, food poisoning or a virus.

NEBULIZER a device for producing a fine spray. Many inhaled drugs are administered in this way, and it is an effective method of delivering a concentrated form of medication e.g. bronchodilators.

NECROSIS death of tissue in a localized area or organ, caused by disease, injury or loss of blood supply.

NEONATAL term meaning relating to the first 28 days of life.

NEOPLASM a new and abnormal growth of cells i.e. a tumour, which may be benign or malignant.

NEPHRITIS inflammation of the KIDNEY, which may be due to one of several causes. Types of nephritis include glomerulonephritis (when the glomerulus is affected), acute nephritis, hereditary nephritis, etc.

NEPHRON see KIDNEY.

NERVE a bundle of nerve fibres comprising NEURONS and glial (supporting) cells (see GLIA), all contained in a fibrous sheath, the perineurium. Motor nerves carry (efferent) impulses in motor neurons from the brain (or spinal cord) to muscles or glands and a sensory nerve carries (afferent) impulses in sensory neurons from sensory organs to the brain or spinal cord. Most large nerves are mixed nerves containing both motor and sensory nerves.

NERVE INJURY nerves may be injured by being severed, pressure may damage a nerve directly or push it against a bone. Damage to a sensory nerve results in a lack of or lessening in sensation, while paralysis of muscles will result from damage to the associated motor nerve.

NERVOUS SYSTEM the complete system of tissues and cells including NERVES, NEURONS, SYNAPSES and receptors (a special cell sensitive to a particular stimulus which then sends an impulse through the nervous system). The nervous system operates through the transmission of impulses that are conducted rapidly to and from muscles, organs etc. It consists of the central nervous system (brain and spinal cord) and the peripheral nervous system that includes the cranial and spinal nerves (see AUTONOMIC NERVOUS SYSTEM).

NEURALGIA strictly, pain in some part or the whole of a nerve (without any physical change in the nerve) but used more widely to encompass pain following the course of a nerve or its branches, whatever the cause. Neuralgia often occurs at the same time each day and is frequently an agonizing pain. It occurs in several forms and is named accordingly, e.g. SCIATICA, trigeminal neuralgia (affecting the face, see TRIGEMINAL NERVE) and intercostal neuralgia (affecting the ribs). Treatment often involves the application of ointments, and the taking of pain-killing drugs. If such treatments do not bring relief, it is possible to freeze the nerve or destroy part of it by surgery.

NEURITIS inflammation of a nerve or nerves which may be due to inflammation from nearby tissues, or a more general condition in which the nerve fibres degenerate. This latter condition (*polyneuritis*) is due to a systemic poison such as alcohol or long-term exposure to solvents such as naphtha.

NEUROMUSCULAR JUNCTION the area of membrane between a muscle cell and a motor NEURON forming a SYNAPSE between the two. Nerve impulses travel down the neuron and each releases *acetylcholine* which depolarizes the enlarged end of the neuron (the motor end plate) slightly. These small depolarizations are totalled until a threshold of -50mV is reached and this results in the production of an 'action potential' that crosses the synapse into the muscle fibre, thereby producing a muscle contraction.

NEURON a nerve cell, vital in the transmission of impulses. Each cell has an enlarged portion (the cell body) from which extends the long, thin axon for carrying impulses away. Shorter, more numerous dendrites receive impulses. The transmission of impulses is faster in axons that are covered in a sheath of MYELIN.

NEUROPATHY any disease that affects the peripheral nerves, whether singly (mononeuropathy) or more generally (polyneuropathy). The symptoms depend upon the type and the nerves affected.

NEUROTRANSMITTER one of several chemical substances released in minute quantities by axon tips into the SYNAPSE to enable a nerve impulse to cross. It diffuses across the space and may depolarize the opposite membrane allowing the production of an action potential (*see* NERVE IMPULSE). Outside the central nervous system *acetylcholine* is a major neurotransmitter, and NORADRENALINE is released in the SYMPATHETIC NERVOUS SYSTEM. Acetylcholine and noradrenaline also operate within the central nervous system as does DOPAMINE, amongst others.

NORADRENALINE (norepine-phrine in U.S.) a NEUROTRANSMITTER of the SYMPATH-ETIC NERVOUS SYSTEM secreted by nerve endings and also the adrenal glands. It is similar to ADRENALINE in structure and function. It increases blood pressure by constricting the vessel, slows the heartbeat, increases breathing both in rate and depth.

NOSE the olfactory organ and also a pathway for air entering the body, by which route it is warmed, filtered and moistened before passing into the lungs. The 'external' nose leads to the NASAL CAVITY which has a mucous membrane with olfactory cells.

NOTIFIABLE DISEASES diseases that must be reported to the health authorities to enable rapid control and monitoring to be undertaken. The list varies between countries but in the U.K. includes acute poliomyeli-tis, AIDS, cholera, dysentery, food poisoning, measles, meningitis, rabies, rubella, scarlet fever, smallpox, tetanus, typhoid fever, viral hepatitis and whooping cough.

OCCIPITAL BONE a bone of the SKULL which is shaped like a saucer and forms the back of the cranium and part of its base. Arising from the base of thin bone are two occipital condyles that articulate with the first cervical vertebrae (the atlas) of the spinal column.

OCCLUSION the closing or blocking of an organ or duct. In dentistry it is the way the teeth meet when the jaws are closed.

OCULOMOTOR NERVE either of a pair of cranial nerves which are involved in eye movements including movement of the eyeball, and alterations in the size of the pupil and lens.

OEDEMA an accumulation of fluid in the body, possibly beneath the skin or in cavities or organs. With an injury the swelling may be localized or more general as in cases of kidney or heart failure. Fluid can collect in the chest cavity, abdomen or lung (PULMONARY OEDEMA). The causes are numerous, e.g. CIRRHOSIS of the liver, heart or kidney failure, starvation, acute NEPHRITIS, allergies or drugs. To alleviate the symptom, the root cause has to be removed. Subcutaneous oedema commonly occurs in women before menstruation, as swollen legs or ankles, but does subside if the legs are rested in a raised position.

OESOPHAGUS the first part of the ALIMENTARY CANAL lying between the PHARYNX and stomach. The mucous membrane lining produces secretions to lubricate food as it passes and the movement of the food to the stomach is achieved by waves of muscular movement called *peristalsis*.

OESTROGEN one of a group of STEROID hormones secreted mainly by the ovaries and to a lesser extent by the adrenal cortex and placenta. (The testes also produce small amounts). Oestrogens control the female secondary sexual characteristics, i.e. enlargement of the breasts, change in the profile of the pelvic girdle, pubic hair growth and deposition of body fat. High levels are produced at ovulation and with PROGESTERONE they regulate the female reproductive cycle.

OLFACTION the sense of smell, *see* NOSE.

OLFACTORY NERVE one of a pair of sensory nerves for smell. It is the first cranial nerve and comprises many fine threads connecting receptors in the mucous membrane of the olfactory area which pass through holes in the skull, fuse to form one fibre and then pass back to the brain.

ONCOGENIC any factor that causes cancer. This may be an organism, a chemical or some environmental condition. Some viruses are oncogenic and have the result of making a normal cell become a cancer cell.

OPIATE one of several drugs, derived from opium and including morphine and codeine. They act by depressing the central nervous system, thus relieving pain and suppressing coughing. Morphine and heroin, its synthetic derivative, are narcotics.

OPPORTUNISTIC an infection that is contracted by someone with a lower resistance than usual. This may be due to drugs or another disease such as DIABETES MELLITUS, cancer or AIDS. In normal circumstances, in a healthy person, the infecting organism would not cause the disease.

OPTIC ATROPHY a deterioration and wasting of the optic disc due to degeneration of fibres in the optic nerve. It may accompany numerous conditions including DIABETES, ARTERIOSCLEROSIS, GLAUCOMA or may be due to a congenital defect, inflammation or injury, or toxic poisoning from alcohol, lead, etc.

OPTIC CHIASMA (OPTIC COMMISSURE) the cross-shaped structure formed from a crossing over of the optic nerves running back from the eyeballs to meet beneath the brain in the midline.

ORGAN any distinct and recognizable unit within the body that is composed of two or more types of tissue and that is responsible for a particular function or functions. Examples are the liver, kidney, heart and brain.

ORTHOPNOEA a severe difficulty in breathing that is so bad that a patient cannot lie and has to sleep in a sitting position. It usually only occurs with serious conditions of the heart and lungs.

OSMOSIS the process whereby solvent molecules (usually water) move through a semi-permeable membrane to the more concentrated solution. Cell membranes function as semi-permeable membranes and osmosis is important in regulating water content in living systems.

OSSICLE the term for a small bone, often applied to those of the middle ear, the auditory ossicles (*see* EAR), that transmit sound to the inner ear from the eardrum.

OSSIFICATION (*or* OSTEOGEN-ESIS) bone formation, which occurs in several stages via special cells called OSTEOBLASTS. Collagen fibres form a network in connective tissue and then a cement of polysaccharide is laid down. Finally, calcium salts are distributed among the cement as tiny crystals. The osteoblasts are enclosed as bone cells (OSTEOCYTES).

OSTEITIS inflammation of bone, caused by damage, infection or bodily disorder. Symptoms include swelling, tenderness, a dull aching sort of pain and redness cover the affected area.

OSTEOARTHRITIS a form of ARTHRITIS involving joint cartilage with accompanying changes in the associated bone. It usually involves the loss of cartilage and the development of OSTEOPHYTES at the bone margins. The function of the joint (most often the thumb, knee and hip) is affected and it becomes painful. The condition may be due to overuse, and affects those past middle age. It also may complicate other joint diseases. Treatment usually involves administering ANALGESICS, possibly anti-inflammatory drugs and the use of corrective or replacement surgery.

OSTEOBLAST a specialized cell responsible for the formation of bone.

OSTEOCHONDRITIS inflammation of bone and cartilage.

OSTEOCHONDROSIS a disease affecting the OSSIFICATION centres of bone in children. It begins with degeneration and NECROSIS but it regenerates and calcifies again.

OSTEOCYTE a bone cell formed from an osteoblast that is no longer active and has become embedded in the matrix of the bone.

OSTEOGENESIS IMPERFECTA (BRITTLE BONE DISEASE) an hereditary disease which results in the bones being unusually fragile and brittle. It may have associated symptoms, namely transparent teeth, unusually mobile joints, dwarfism, etc. It may be due to a disorder involving collagen, but there is little that can be done in treatment.

OSTEOMALACIA a softening of the bones, and the adult equivalent of RICKETS, which is due to a lack of Vitamin D. This vitamin is obtained from the diet and is produced on exposure to sunlight, and it is necessary for the uptake of calcium from food.

OSTEOMYELITIS bone marrow inflammation caused by infection. This may happen after a compound fracture or during bone surgery. It produces pain, swelling and fever and high doses of antibiotics are necessary.

OSTEOPHYTE bony projections that occur near joints or interverte-bral discs where cartilage has degenerated or been destroyed (*see* OSTEOARTHRITIS). Osteophytes may in any case occur with increasing age with or without loss of cartilage.

OSTEOPOROSIS a loss of bone tissue due to it being resorbed, resulting in bones that become brittle and likely to fracture. It is common in menopausal women and results from long-term steroid therapy. It is also a feature of CUSHING'S SYNDROME. Hormone replacement therapy is a treatment available to women.

OSTEOSARCOMA the commonest and most malignant bone tumour that is found most in older children. The femur is usually affected but metastases are common (*see* METASTASIS). It produces pain and swelling and although amputation used to be the standard treatment, surgery is now possible, with replacement of the diseased bone and associated chemotherapy and/or radiotherapy. It remains, nevertheless, a serious cancer with a relatively poor survival rate.

OSTEOSCLEROSIS a condition in which the density of bone tissue increases abnormally. It is due to tumour, infection or poor blood supply and may be due to an abnormality involving osteoclasts, cells that resorb calcified bone.

OTITIS inflammation of the ear. This may take several forms depending upon the exact location which produces diverse symptoms e.g. inflammation of the inner ear (*otitis interna*), affects balance, causing vertigo and vomiting while *otitis media* is usually a bacterial infection of the middle ear resulting in severe pain, and a fever requiring immediate antibiotic treatment. *Secretory otitis media* is otherwise known as GLUE EAR.

OTOSCLEROSIS the hereditary condition in which there is overgrowth of bone in the inner ear which restricts and then stops sound being conducted to the inner EAR from the middle ear. The person affected becomes progressively more deaf, often beginning with TINNITUS, but surgery is effective.

OVARY the reproductive organ of females which produces eggs (ova) and hormones (mainly OESTROGEN and PROGESTERONE). There are two ovaries, each the size of an almond, on either side of the uterus and each contains numerous Graafian FOLLICLES in which the eggs develop. At OVULATION an egg is released from a follicle. The follicles secrete oestrogen and progesterone which regulate the menstrual cycle and the uterus during pregnancy.

OVULATION the release of an egg from an OVARY (i.e. from a mature Graafian follicle) which then moves down the FALLOPIAN TUBE to the uterus. Ovulation is brought about by secretion of *luteinizing hormone*

secreted by the anterior PITUITARY GLAND.

OVUM (*plural* OVA) the mature, unfertilized female reproductive cell which is roughly spherical with an outer membrane and a single nucleus.

P

PALLIATIVE a medicine or treatment that is given to effect some relief from symptoms, if only temporarily, but does not cure the ailment. This is often the case in the treatment of cancer.

PALLOR an abnormal paleness of skin because of a reduced blood flow, or a lack of the normal pigments. It may be due directly to ANAEMIA or SHOCK to spending an excessive amount of time indoors.

PALPATION examination of the surface of the body by carefully feeling with hands and fingertips. It is often possible to distinguish between solid lumps or swelling and cystic swellings.

PALPITATION when the heart beats noticeably or irregularly and the person becomes aware of it. The heartbeat is not normally noticed but with fear, emotion or exercise it may be felt, unpleasantly so. Palpitations may also be due to neuroses, ARRHYTHMIA, heart disease and a common cause is too much tea, coffee, alcohol or smoking. Where an excess is the cause (tea, coffee etc.) this can be eliminated. For disease-associated palpitations, drugs can be used for control.

PALSY the term used formerly for paralysis and retained for the names of some conditions.

PANCREAS a gland with both ENDOCRINE and exocrine functions. It is located between the DUODENUM and

SPLEEN, behind the stomach, and is about 15cm long. There are two types of cells producing secretions, the *acini* which produce pancreatic juice which goes to the intestine via a system of ducts. This contains an alkaline mixture of salt and enzymes - trypsin and chymotrypsin to digest proteins, amylase to break down starch and lipase to aid digestion of fats. The second cell types are in the ISLETS OF LANGERHANS and these produce two hormones, INSULIN and GLUCAGON, secreted directly into the blood for control of sugar levels (*see also* DIABETES MELLITUS, HYPO- and HYPERGLYCAEMIA).

PANCREATITIS inflammation of the PANCREAS, occurring in several forms, but often associated with gallstones or alcoholism. Any bout of the condition that interferes with the function of the pancreas may lead to DIABETES and MALABSORPTION.

PAPILLA any small protuberance such as the papillae on the tongue.

PAPILLOMA usually benign growths on the skin surface or mucous membrane e.g. WARTS.

PARALYSIS muscle weakness or total loss of muscle movement which varies depending upon the causal disease and its effect on the brain. Various descriptive terms are used to qualify the parts of the body affected, thus hemiplegia affects one side of the body (*see also* DIPLEGIA, PARAPLEGIA, QUADRIPLEGIA). Paralysis is really a symptom of another condition or disease e.g. brain disease such as a cerebral haemorrhage or THROMBOSIS causing hemiplegia; disease or injury of the spinal cord leading to paraplegia; and POLIOMYELITIS (infantile paralysis). In addition there is the paralysis associated with MOTOR NEURONE DISEASE.

PARAPLEGIA PARALYSIS of the legs. It may be caused by injury or disease of the spinal cord and often

bladder and rectum are also affected.

PARASITE any organism that obtains its nutrients by living in or on the body of another organism (the *host*). The extent to which the host is damaged by the parasite ranges from virtually no effect to, in extreme cases, death. Parasites in humans include worms, viruses, fungi, etc.

PARASYMPATHETIC NERVOUS SYSTEM one of the two parts of the AUTONOMIC NERVOUS SYSTEM that acts antagonistically with the SYMPATHETIC NERVOUS SYSTEM. The parasympathetic nerves originate from the brain and lower portion of the spinal cord (sacral region). The AXONS of this system tend to be longer than sympathetic nerves and SYNAPSES with other neurons are close to the target organ. The parasympathetic system contracts the bladder, decreases heart rate, stimulates the sex organs, promotes digestion, etc.

PARATHYROID GLANDS four small glands located behind or within the thyroid gland, that control the metabolism of calcium and phosphorus (as phosphate) in the body. The hormone responsible, parathormone (or simply parathyroid hormone) is produced and released by the glands. A deficiency of the hormone leads to lower levels of calcium in the blood with a relative increase in phosphorus. This produces tetany, a condition involving muscular spasms, which can be treated by injection. This is also known as *hypoparathyroidism* and is often due to removal or injury of the glands during thyroidectomy. If the hormone is at high levels calcium is transferred from bones to the blood, causing weakness and susceptibility to breaks.

PAROTID GLAND one of a pair of salivary glands situated in front of each ear and opening inside on the cheek near the second last molar of the upper jaw.

PAROTITIS inflammation of the PAROTID GLAND, which as epidemic or infectious parotitis is called MUMPS.

PAROXYSM a sudden attack. A term used especially about convulsions.

PATELLA the kneecap. An almost flat bone, shaped somewhat like an oyster shell, that lies in front of the knee in the tendon of the thigh muscle.

PATELLAR REFLEX see REFLEX ACTION.

PATHOGEN the term applied to an organism that causes disease. Most pathogens affecting humans are bacteria and viruses.

PECTORAL the descriptive term for anything relating to the chest.

PECTORAL GIRDLE (or shoulder girdle) the skeletal structure to which the bones of the upper limbs are attached. It is composed of two shoulder blades (SCAPULAE) and two collar bones (CLAVICLES) attached to the vertebral column and breastbone (sternum) respectively.

PELVIC GIRDLE (or hip girdle) the skeletal structure to which the bones of the lower limbs are attached. It is made up of the two hip bones, each comprising the ilium, pubis and ischium, fused together.

PENIS the male organ through which the URETHRA passes, carrying urine or semen. It is made up of tissue that is filled with blood during sexual arousal, producing an erection which enables penetration of the vagina and ejaculation of semen. The glans is the end part normally covered by the FORESKIN (prepuce).

PEPTIC ULCER an ulcer in the stomach (GASTRIC ULCER), oesophagus, duodenum (DUODENAL ULCER), or JEJUNUM. It is caused by a break in the mucosal lining due to the action of acid and pepsin (an enzyme active in protein breakdown) either because of their high concentrations or due to other factors affecting the mucosal protective mechanisms.

PERFORATION when a hole forms in a hollow organ, tissue or tube, e.g. the stomach, eardrum etc. In particular, it is a serious development of an ulcer in the stomach or bowels because on perforation the intestine contents, with bacteria, enter the peritoneal (see PERITONEUM) cavity causing PERITONITIS. This is accompanied by severe pain and shock and usually corrective surgery is required.

PERICARDITIS inflammation of the PERICARDIUM. It may be due to URAEMIA, cancer or viral infection and produces fever, chest pain and possible accumulation of fluid.

PERICARDIUM the smooth membrane surrounding the heart. The outer *fibrous* part covers the heart and is connected to the large vessels coming out of the heart. The inner *serous* part is a closed SEROUS MEMBRANE attached both to the fibrous pericardium and the heart wall. Some fluid in the resulting sac enables smooth movement as the heart beats.

PERINATAL MORTALITY foetal deaths after week 28 of pregnancy and newborn deaths during the first week or two of life. The main causes of perinatal mortality are brain injuries during birth, congenital defects and lack of oxygen in the final stages of pregnancy (called *antepartum anoxia*). Perinatal *deaths* are due to complications involving the placenta, congenital defects and birth asphyxia.

PERINEUM the area of the body between anus and urethral opening.

PERIODONTAL descriptive term relating to the tissues surrounding the teeth.

PERIPHERAL NERVOUS SYSTEM those parts of the nervous system excluding the central nervous system (brain and spinal cord). It comprises the afferent (sensory) and efferent (motor) cells which include

12 pairs of cranial nerves and 31 pairs of spinal nerves. The motor nervous system then comprises the somatic nervous system carrying impulses to the skeletal muscles, and the autonomic nervous system which is further divided into the sympathetic and the parasympathetic nervous system (*see individual entries*).

PERIPHERAL NEURITIS inflammation of the nerves of the peripheral nervous system.

PERITONEUM the SEROUS MEMBRANE that lines the abdominal cavity. That lining the abdomen walls is the *parietal* peritoneum while the *visceral* peritoneum covers the organs. The folds of peritoneum from one organ to another are given special names, e.g. MESENTERY. Both are continuous and form a closed sac at the back of the abdomen in the male, while in the female there is an opening from the Fallopian tube on either side.

PERITONITIS inflammation of the peritoneum. It may be caused by a primary infection due to bacteria in the bloodstream (e.g. tuberculous peritonitis) resulting in pain and swelling, fever and weight loss. Secondary infection results from entry into the abdominal cavity of bacteria and irritants (e.g. digestive juices) from a perforated or ruptured organ e.g. duodenum or stomach. This produces severe pain and shock and surgery is often necessary.

PERSPIRATION (*or* **SWEAT**) the excretion from millions of tiny sweat glands in the skin. Sweat that evaporates from the skin immediately is *insensible*, while that forming drops is *sensible perspiration*. Sweat is produced in two types of sweat glands. The *eccrine* glands are found mainly on the soles of the feet and palms of the hands. The *apocrine* glands are in the armpits, around the anus and genitalia and sweat is produced in response to stimuli such as fear and sexual arousal. The major function of sweating, however, is the regulation of body temperature.

PERTUSSIS *see* **WHOOPING COUGH**.

PETIT MAL the lesser type of epileptic seizure which is IDIOPATHIC. It consists of brief periods (seconds) of unconsciousness when the eyes stare blankly but posture is maintained. Children suffering frequently may have learning difficulties but the condition may disappear in adult life.

PHAGOCYTOSIS *see* **LEUCO-CYTE**.

PHALLUS the penis, or a penis-like object. Also the term used for the embryonic penis before the final development of the urethral duct.

PHARYNGITIS inflammation of the PHARYNX and therefore throat, commonly due to a virus, and resulting in a sore throat. It is often associated with TONSILLITIS.

PHARYNX the region extending from the beginning of the oesophagus up to the base of the skull at the cavity into which nose and mouth open. It is muscular, with a mucous membrane and acts as the route for both food (to the oesophagus) and air (to the larynx). The EUSTACHIAN TUBES open from the upper part of the pharynx.

PHIMOSIS a condition in which the edge of the FORESKIN is narrowed and cannot be drawn back over the glans of the PENIS. To avoid inflammation and an exacerbation of the problem, circumcision may be necessary.

PHLEBITIS inflammation of a vein. This commonly occurs as a complication of VARICOSE VEINS, producing pain and a hot feeling around the vein, with possible THROMBOSIS development. Drugs and elastic support are used in treatment.

PHLEBOTHROMBOSIS the obstruction of a vein by a blood clot, common in the deep veins of the leg (in particular the calf) and resulting from heart failure, pregnancy, injury and surgery, which may change the clotting factors in the blood. The affected leg may swell and there is the danger that the clot may move, creating a PULMONARY EMBOLISM.

PHOBIA an anxiety disorder and irrational fear of certain objects, animals, situations, events, etc. Avoiding the situation can lead to significant disruption, restriction of normal life or even suffering. There is a variety of phobias including animal, specific and social phobias and treatment involves through behaviour therapy.

PHONATION the production of speech sounds.

PHOTOPHOBIA an atypical sensitivity to light. Exposure produces discomfort and actions to evade the light source. The condition may be associated with medications, or migraine, meningitis, etc.

PHRENIC NERVE the nerve to the muscles of the DIAPHRAGM, arising from the 3rd, 4th and 5th cervical spinal nerves.

PHYSICAL concerning the body as opposed to the mind.

PIA MATER *see* BRAIN and MENINGES.

PIGMENT an organic colouring agent e.g. the blood pigment HAEMOGLOBIN, BILE pigments, rhodopsin (found in the RODS of the RETINA) and MELANIN.

PILES *see* HAEMORRHOIDS.

PILUS a hair or structure like a hair.

PIMPLES (papules) small swellings on the skin that are inflamed and may contain pus. The cause is often infection of a pore that is blocked with fatty secretions from the SEBACEOUS GLANDS. On the face, the condition is called ACNE.

PITUITARY GLAND (*or* **HYPOPHYSIS**) a small, but very important endocrine gland at the base of the HYPOTHALAMUS. It has two lobes, the anterior *adenohypophysis*

and the posterior *neurohypophysis*. The pituitary secretes hormones that control many functions and is itself controlled by hormonal secretions from the hypothalamus. The neurohypophysis stores and releases peptide hormones produced in the hypothalamus namely OXYTOCIN and VASOPRESSIN. The adenohypophysis secretes GROWTH HORMONE, GONADOTROPHIN, prolactin (involved in stimulating lactation), ACTH and THYROID stimulating hormones.

PLACENTA the organ attaching the embryo to the UTERUS. It is a temporary feature comprising maternal and embryonic tissues and it allows oxygen and nutrients to pass from the mother's blood to the embryo's blood. There is, however, no direct contact of blood supplies. The embryo also receives salt, glucose, amino acids, some peptides and antibodies, fats and vitamins. Waste molecules from the embryo are removed by diffusion into the maternal circulation. It also stores GLYCOGEN for conversion to glucose if required and secretes hormones to regulate the pregnancy. It is expelled after birth.

PLANTAR descriptive term meaning relating to the sole of the foot.

PLAQUE a surface layer on teeth formed from bacteria and food debris and later, calcium salts.

PLASMA a light-coloured fluid component of BLOOD and in which the various cells are suspended. It contains inorganic salts with protein and some trace substances. One protein present is FIBRINOGEN.

PLATELET (*or* **THROMBO-CYTE**) a disc like structure in the blood involved in the halting of bleeding.

PLEURA the SEROUS MEMBRANE that covers the lungs (*visceral*) and the inside of the chest wall (*parietal*). The membranes have a smooth surface which is moistened to allow them to slide over each other.

PLEURAL CAVITY the small space between the PLEURA which slide over each other when breathing in and out. Should gas or fluid enter the cavity due to infection or injury the space increases and may hinder breathing.

PLEURISY (or PLEURITIS) inflammation of the PLEURA resulting in pain from deep breathing, and resulting shortness of breath. There is a typical frictional rub heard through a stethoscope. Pleurisy is often due to pneumonia in the adjacent lung and is always associated with disease in the lung, diaphragm, chest wall or abdomen e.g. tuberculosis, abscesses, bronchial carcinoma etc.

PLEXUS a network formed from intersecting nerves and/or blood vessels, or lymphatic vessels.

PNEUMONIA a bacterial infection of the lungs resulting in inflammation and filling of the ALVEOLI with pus and fluid. As a result the lung becomes solid and air cannot enter. The symptoms vary depending upon how much of the lung is unavailable for respiration, but commonly there will be chest pain, coughing, breathlessness, fever and possibly CYANOSIS. Pneumonia may be caused by several bacteria, viruses or fungi, but bacterial infection is commonest. Bronchopneumonia affects the bronchi and bronchioles; lobar pneumonia the whole lobes of the lung(s). Antibiotic treatment is usually effective although it helps to know which is the infecting organism, to provide the most specific treatment. (*See also* VIRAL PNEUMONIA).

PNEUMONITIS inflammation of the lungs by chemical or physical agents.

PNEUMOTHORAX air in the PLEURAL CAVITY, which enters via a wound in the chest wall or lung. When this happens, the lung collapses but if the air is absorbed from the pleural cavity the lung reinflates.

POCK a small eruption on the skin, which may contain pus, typical of chickenpox and smallpox.

POLIOMYELITIS (or INFAN- TILE PARALYSIS, POLIO) an infectious disease, caused by a virus, which attacks the central nervous system. The virus is taken in by mouth, passes through the digestive system, is excreted in the faeces and hands may be contaminated, leading to further spread. The incubation period is 7 to 12 days and there are several types of condition, depending upon the severity of the attack. In some cases the symptoms resemble a stomach upset or influenza; in others there is in addition some stiffness of muscles. Paralytic poliomyelitis is less common, resulting in muscle weakness and paralysis while the most serious cases involve breathing when the diaphragm and related muscles are affected (bulbar poliomyelitis). Immunization is highly effective and the disease has almost been eradicated in most countries. However, booster doses are advisable when visiting countries with a high incidence of the disease.

POLYDIPSIA an intense thirst, abnormally so. It is a characteristic symptom of DIABETES MELLITUS and certain other diseases.

POLYP a growth from a mucous membrane and attached to it by a stalk. Most are benign but may cause obstructions or infections. They commonly occur in the sinuses, nose, or possibly the bladder or bowels. Their removal is usually straightforward, unless a more extensive operation proves necessary to reach the affected organ.

POLYURIA the passing of a larger

than normal quantity of urine which is also usually pale in colour. It may be due merely to a large fluid intake, or to a condition such as DIABETES, or a kidney disorder.

PONS tissue that joins parts of an organ, e.g. the *pons Varolii*, a part of the brainstem links various parts of the brain including the medulla oblongata and thalamus.

PORE a small opening, e.g. sweat pores.

PORTAL VEIN a vein within the hepatic portal system that carries blood to the liver from other abdominal organs (stomach, spleen, intestine, etc.). It is atypical in that it does not take blood directly to the heart but ends in a capillary network.

POSSETTING the term for the normal habit of some quite healthy babies to regurgitate small amounts of a recently-taken meal.

POULTICE (*or* **FOMENTATION**) hot, moist material applied to the body to soften the skin, soothe irritations, ease pain or increase the circulation locally.

POX pus-filled pimples as in chickenpox or smallpox. Also the small pit-like depressions that are scars of smallpox.

PRECANCEROUS any condition that is not malignant but is known will become so if left untreated.

PRE-ECLAMPSIA the development of high blood pressure in pregnancy, sometimes with OEDEMA which unless treated may result in ECLAMPSIA.

PREGNANCY the period of time, lasting approximately 280 days from the first day of the last menstrual period, during which a woman carries a developing foetus. Signs of a pregnancy include cessation of menstruation, increase in size of the breasts, MORNING SICKNESS, and later in the pregnancy the obvious sign of enlargement of the abdomen. A foetal heart beat and movements also follow later. Many of these changes are hormone-controlled, by progesterone (from the OVARY and PLACENTA).

PREMOLAR two teeth between the canines and molars on each side of the jaw.

PREPUCE *see* FORESKIN.

PRESENTATION the point, during LABOUR, at which some part of the foetus lies at the mouth of the womb. In the majority of cases the head presents, but *see* BREECH PRESENTATION.

PRESSURE SORES *see* BED SORES.

PRICKLY HEAT (heat rash or miliaria) an itchy rash due to small red spots which are minute vesicles caused by the blocking of sweat or sebaceous glands in the skin. Scratching may produce infection but the condition itself is not serious.

PROGESTERONE a steroid hormone that is vital in pregnancy. It is produced by the CORPUS LUTEUM of the OVARY when the lining of the uterus is prepared for the implanting of an egg cell. Progesterone is secreted under the control of other hormones (prolactin from the anterior PITUITARY, and luteinizing hormone also from the pituitary which stimulates ovulation and formation of the corpus luteum) until the placenta adopts this role later in the pregnancy. The function of progesterone is to maintain the uterus and ensure no further eggs are produced. Small amounts of this hormone are also produced by the testes.

PROGNOSIS a forecast of the likely outcome of a disease, based upon the patient's condition and the course of the disease in other patients at other times.

PROLAPSE a moving down of an organ or tissue from its normal position due to the supporting tissues weakening. This may happen to the lower end of the bowel (in children)

163   **PULMONARY HYPERTENSION**

or the uterus and vagina in women
who have sustained some sort of
injury during childbirth. In the latter
case prolapse may result in the
uterus itself showing on the outside.
Surgery can shorten the supporting
ligaments and narrow the vaginal
opening.

**PROLAPSED INTERVERTE-
BRAL DISC (SLIPPED DISC)** the
intervertebral disc provides
cushioning for the brain and spinal
cord and is composed of an outer
fibrous layer over a pulpy centre. A
slipped disc is caused by the inner
layer being pushed through the
fibrous layer to impinge upon
nerves, causing pain (commonly
lumbago or sciatica). The prolapse
usually occurs during sudden
twisting or bending of the backbone
and is more likely to occur during
middle age. Treatment involves bed
rest on a flat, firm surface, probably
with manipulation and physiotherapy
at a later stage. If absolutely
necessary, the disc can be removed,
but this is now less common.

PRONE lying face downwards.

PROPHYLACTIC some treatment
or action that is taken to avoid
disease or a condition, e.g. taking a
medication to prevent angina.

PROSTAGLANDIN (PG) a group
of compounds derived from essential
fatty acids that act in a way that is
similar to hormones. They are found
in most body tissues (but especially
semen) where they are released as
local regulators (in the uterus, brain,
lungs, etc.). A number have been
identified, two of which act
antagonistically on blood vessels.
PGE causing dilation, PGF
constriction. Certain prostaglandins
cause uterine contraction in labour,
and others are involved in the body's
defence mechanisms.

PROSTATE GLAND a gland in the
male reproductive system which is
located below the bladder, opening

into the URETHRA. Upon ejaculation, it
secretes an alkaline fluid into the
semen which aids sperm motility. In
older men, the gland may become
enlarged, causing problems with
urination.

PROSTHESES (*singular*
PROSTHESIS) artificial devices
fitted to the body, ranging from
dentures to hearing aids, pacemakers
and artificial limbs.

PRURITUS another term for
itching, of whatever origin.

PSORIASIS a chronic skin disease
for which the cause is unknown and
the treatment is palliative. The
affected skin appears as itchy, scaly
red areas, starting usually around the
elbows and knees. It often runs in
families and may be associated with
anxiety, commencing usually in
childhood or adolescence. Treatment
involves the use of ointments and
creams with some drugs and
vitamin A.

PUBIS one of three bones, and the
most anterior, that makes up each
half of the pelvic girdle.

PULMONARY relating to the
lungs.

PULMONARY EMBOLISM a
condition involving the blocking of
the pulmonary artery or a branch of
it by an EMBOLUS (usually a blood
clot). The clot usually originates
from PHLEBOTHROMBOSIS of the leg.
The seriousness of the attack relates
to the size of the clot. Large
pulmonary emboli can be immediately fatal. Smaller ones may cause
death of parts of the lung, PLEURISY
and coughing up of blood.
Anticoagulant drugs are used in
minor cases; streptokinase may be
used to dissolve the clot or
immediate surgery may be
necessary. Several embolisms may
produce PULMONARY HYPERTENSION.

PULMONARY HYPERTENSION
an increase in blood pressure in the
pulmonary artery due to increased

resistance to the flow of blood. The cause is usually disease of the lung (such as BRONCHITIS, EMPHYSEMA, *see also* PULMONARY EMBOLISM) and the result is that the pressure increases in the right ventricle, enlarging it, producing pain with the possibility of heart failure.

PULSE the regular expansion and contraction of an artery as a fluid wave of blood passes along, originating with the contraction of the heart muscle and blood leaving the left ventricle. It is detected on arteries near the surface, e.g. the radial artery on the wrist and decreases with a reduction in the size of artery so that the capillaries are under a steady pressure (hence the reason why venous flow is also steady).

PUPIL the circular opening in the IRIS which permits light into the lens in the EYE.

PUS the liquid found at an infected site (abscess, ulcer, etc.). It is coloured white, yellow or greenish and consists of dead white blood cells, living and dead bacteria and dead tissue.

PYELITIS inflammation of part of the kidney, the pelvis. (This is the area from which urine drains into the ureter). The cause is usually a bacterial infection (commonly *E. coli*) and sometimes occurs as a complication of pregnancy. The symptoms include pain in the loins, high temperature, loss of weight, but it does respond to antibiotics. It is usually the case that the infection is not limited to the pelvis but all the kidney hence a more accurate term is *pyelonephritis*.

PYLORIC STENOSIS a narrowing of the PYLORUS which limits the movement of food from the stomach to the duodenum, resulting in vomiting. It may be accompanied by distension and peristalsis of the stomach, visible through the

abdominal wall. A continuation of the condition causes weight loss and dehydration. It is often due to an ulcer or cancer near the pylorus which requires surgery.

PYLORUS the lower end of the stomach where food passes into the duodenum and at which there is a ring of muscle, the *pyloric sphincter*.

PYREXIA another term for FEVER.

QUADRICEPS the large thigh muscle, which is divided into four distinct parts, and is responsible for movements of the knee joint.

QUADRIPLEGIA paralysis of all four limbs of the body.

QUARANTINE a period of time in which a person (or animal) who has, or is suspected of having, an infectious disease is isolated from others to prevent the spread of the infection.

QUICKENING the first movements of a baby in the womb which are perceived by the mother usually around the fourth month of pregnancy.

QUINSY the medical name for this condition is *pentonsillar abscess* and it is a complication of TONSILLITIS. A pus-filled abscess occurs near the tonsil, causing great difficulty in swallowing, and this may require surgical lancing.

R

RABIES a very severe and fatal disease affecting the central nervous system which occurs in dogs, wolves, cats and other carniverous animals. Human beings are infected through the bite of a *rabid* animal. The onset of symptoms varies from ten days to up to a year from the time of being bitten. Characteristically, the person becomes irritable and depressed, swallowing and breathing difficulties develop, there are periods of great mental excitement, increased salivation and muscular spasms of the throat. Eventually, even the sight of water causes severe muscular spasms, convulsions and paralysis, and death follows within about four days. Treatment consists of thorough cleansing of the bite and injections of rabies vaccine, antiserum and immunoglobulin. As the UK is currently free of rabies, vigilant quarantine and other regulations involving the movement of animals, are in force.

RADIUS the shorter outer bone of the forearm the other being the *ulna*.

RASH an eruption of the skin which is usually short-lived and consists of reddened, perhaps itchy area or raised red spots.

RECTUM the final portion of the large intestine between the colon and anal canal in which faeces are stored prior to elimination.

RED BLOOD CELL *see* ERYTHROCYTE.

REFERRED PAIN (SYNALGIA) pain felt in another part of the body at a distance from the site at which it might be expected. An example is certain heart conditions which cause pain in the left arm and fingers. The condition arises because some sensory nerves share common routes in the central nervous system hence stimulation of one causes an effect in another.

REFLEX ACTION an unconscious movement which is brought about by relatively simple nervous circuits in the central nervous system. In its simplest form it involves a single *reflex arc* of one receptor and

sensory nerve which forms a *synapse* in the BRAIN or SPINAL cord with a motor nerve which then transmits the impulse to a muscle or gland to bring about a response. However some reflex actions are more complicated than this, involving several neurones. Examples are the *plantar reflex* of the toes, when the sole of the foot is stroked, the *knee jerk reflex* and the reflex pupil of the eye which contracts suddenly when a light is directed upon its surface. The presence or absence of reflexes give an indication of the condition of the nervous system and are pointers to the presence or absence of disease or damage.

REGURGITATION the bringing up of swallowed undigested food from the stomach to the mouth (*see also* POSSETTING). The term is also used to describe the backward flow of blood in the heart if one or more valves is diseased and defective.

RELAPSE the return of the symptoms of a disease from which a person had apparently recovered or was in the process of recovery.

RENAL describing or relating to the kidneys.

REPETITIVE STRAIN INJURY *see* TENDINITIS.

REPRODUCTIVE SYSTEM the name given to all the organs involved in reproduction. In males these comprise the testes, vasa deferentia, prostate gland, seminal vesicles, urethra and penis. In females, the reproductive system consists of the ovaries, Fallopian tubes, womb (uterus), vagina and vulva (*see individual entries*).

RESPIRATION the whole process by which air is drawn into and out of the lungs during which oxygen is absorbed into the bloodstream and carbon dioxide and water are given off. *External respiration* is the actual process of breathing and the exchange of gases which takes place in the lungs. *Internal respiration* is the process by which oxygen is given up from the blood circulation to the tissues, in all parts of the body, and carbon dioxide is taken up to be transported back to the lungs and eliminated.

The process of drawing air into the lungs is known as *inhalation* or *inspiration* and expelling it out as *exhalation* or *expiration*. The rate at which this occurs is known as the *respiratory rate* and it is about 18 times a minute in a static healthy adult.

RESPIRATOR one of a number of different devices used to assist or take over RESPIRATION, especially when the muscles which should normally be involved are paralysed, as in some forms of POLIOMYELITIS.

RESPIRATORY DISTRESS SYNDROME this usually refers to a condition arising in newborn babies, especially those which are premature, being particularly common in infants born between 32-37 weeks gestation. It is also known as *hyaline membrane disease* and is characterized by rapid shallow laboured breathing. It arises because the lungs are not properly expanded and lack a substance (known as surfactant) necessary to bring their expansion about.

Adults may suffer from *adult respiratory distress syndrome* in which there is PULMONARY OEDEMA and a high mortality rate.

RESPIRATORY SYNCITIAL VIRUS generally called RS Virus, this is the main cause of BRONCHIOLITIS and pneumonia in babies under the age of 6 months

RESPIRATORY SYSTEM all the organs and tissues involved in RESPIRATION including the nose, pharynx, larynx, trachea, bronchi, bronchioles, lungs and diaphragm, along with the muscles which bring about respiratory movements.

RESUSCITATION reviving a person in whom heart beat and breathing has ceased. SEE ARTIFICIAL RESPIRATION and CARDIAC MASSAGE.

RETINA the layer which lines the interior of the eye. The retina itself consists of two layers the inner one next to the cavity of the eyeball containing the light-sensitive cells, the RODS and CONES, and also nerve fibres. This layer receives light directed onto its surface by the lens. The outer layer of the retina next to the *choroid* contains pigmented cells which prevent the passage of light (*See also* EYE).

RETROVIRUS a type of virus containing RNA (ribonucleic acid) which is able to introduce its genetic material into the DNA of body cells. These viruses are suspected causal agents in the development of certain cancers.

RHESUS FACTOR *see* BLOOD GROUP.

RHEUMATIC FEVER a severe disease affecting children and young adults which is a complication of upper respiratory tract infection with bacteria known as *Haemolytic streptococci*. The symptoms include fever, joint pain and ARTHRITIS which progresses from joint to joint, a characteristic red rash known as *Erythema marginatum* and also painless nodules which develop beneath the skin over bony protuberances such as the elbow, knee and back of the wrist. In addition there is chorea and inflammation of the heart including the muscle, valves and membranes. The condition may lead to rheumatic heart disease in which there is scarring and inflammation of heart structures. There is sometimes a need for heart valves to be replaced in later life.

RHEUMATISM a general term used to describe aches and pains in joints and muscles.

RHEUMATOID ARTHRITIS the

second most common form of joint disease after OSTEOARTHRITIS which usually affects the feet, ankles, fingers and wrists. The condition is diagnosed by means of X-rays which show a typical pattern of changes around the inflamed joints known as *rheumatoid erosions*. At first there is swelling of the joint and inflammation of the SYNOVIAL MEMBRANE (the membranous sac which surrounds the joint), followed by erosion and loss of cartilage and bone. In addition, a blood test reveals the presence of *serum rheumatoid factor antibody* which is characteristic of this condition. The condition varies greatly in its degree of severity but at its worst can be progressive and seriously disabling. In other people, after an initial active phase, there may be a long period of remission. A number of different drugs are used to treat the disease including analgesics and anti-inflammatory agents.

RHINITIS inflammation of the mucous membrane of the nose such as occurs with colds and allergic reactions.

RIBS 12 pairs of thin, slightly twisted and curved bones which form the thoracic rib cage which protects the lungs and heart. The *true ribs* are the first seven pairs which are each connected to the STERNUM at the front by a costal CARTILAGE. The *false ribs* are the next three pairs are indirectly connected to the sternum as each is attached by its cartilage to the rib above. The *floating ribs* are the last two pairs which are unattached and end freely in the muscle of the thoracic wall. At the backbone, the head of each rib articulates with one of the 12 thoracic vertebrae.

RIGOR a sudden bout of shivering and feeling of coldness which often accompanies the start of a fever.

RIGOR MORTIS the stiffening of the body that occurs within eight hours of death due to chemical changes in the muscles.

RINGWORM an infection caused by various species of fungi and is known medically as Tinea. It is classified according to the area affected e.g. *Tinea capitis* which is ringworm of the scalp. Other areas affected are the beard, groin, (dhobie itch), nails and feet (athletes foot). The infection is slightly raised, itchy and with a ring-like appearance. It is highly contagious and the commonest form is athletes foot which usually begins between the toes.

ROD one of the two types of light sensitive cell present in the RETINA of the EYE. The rods enable vision in dim light due to a pigment called *rhodopsin (visual purple)*. This pigment degenerates or bleaches when light is present and regenerates during darkness. In bright light all the pigment bleaches and the rods cannot function. Bleaching of the pigment gives rise to nerve impulses which are sent to the brain and interpreted.

ROSACEA a disease of the skin of the face characterized by a red, flushed appearance and enlargement of the SEBACEOUS GLANDS in the skin. The nose may also enlarge and look red and lumpy (rhinophyma). The cause is unknown but may be aggravated by certain foods or drinks such as an excess of alcohol. Treatment is by means of *tetracycline drugs*.

ROSEOLA any rose-coloured rash such as accompanies various infectious diseases e.g. measles.

ROTAVIRUS one of a number of viruses which commonly cause gastro-enteritis and diarrhoea in young children under the age of 6 years. They infect the lining cells of the SMALL INTESTINE.

RUBELLA *see* GERMAN MEASLES.

RUPTURE the bursting open of an organ, tissue or structure, e.g. ruptured

APPENDIX. Also, a popular name for a HERNIA.

S

SAC a structure resembling a bag, e.g. the lungs.

SACRAL NERVES nerves that serve the legs, anal and genital region and which originate from the sacral area of the spinal column. There are five pairs of sacral nerves.

SACRAL VERTEBRAE the five vertebrae that are fused together form the SACRUM.

SACRUM the lower part of the spinal column comprising five fused vertebrae (SACRAL VERTEBRAE) in a triangular shape. The sacrum forms the back wall of the pelvis and articulates with the coccyx below, lumbar vertebrae above and the hips to the sides.

SALIVA an alkaline liquid present in the mouth to keep the mouth moist, aid swallowing of food and through the presence of amylase enzymes (ptyalin) to digest starch. It is secreted by the SALIVARY GLANDS and in addition to ptyalin, contains water, mucus and buffers (to minimise changes in acidity).

SALIVARY GLANDS three pairs of glands; parotid, submandibular and sublingual, that produce saliva. The stimulus to produce saliva can be the taste, smell, sight or even thought of food.

SALMONELLA INFECTIONS FOOD POISONING due to Salmonella, a genus of Gram-negative (see GRAM'S STAIN) rodlike bacteria.

SARCOMA see CANCER.

SCALDS see BURNS.

SCALP the covering of the skull around the top of the head which comprises several layers, from the skin with hair on the outside through fat and fibrous tissue to another fibrous layer (the pericranium) that is attached closely to the skull.

SCALPEL a small surgical knife with renewable blades, used for cutting tissues.

SCAN examination of the body using one of a number of techniques, such as computerized tomography AND ultrasonography (see ULTRA-SOUND).

SCAPHOID BONE a bone of the wrist, the outside one on the thumb side of the hand.

SCAPULA the shoulder blade. A triangular bone and one of a pair forming the shoulder girdle.

SCAR the mark left after a wound heals. It is due to the damaged tissues not repairing completely, and being replaced by a fibrous connective tissue.

SCARLET FEVER an infectious disease, mainly of childhood, caused by the bacterium Streptococcus. Symptoms show after a few days and include sickness, sore throat, fever and a scarlet rash that may be widespread. Antibiotics are effective and also prevent any complications e.g. inflammation of the kidneys.

SCIATICA pain in the sciatic nerve, and therefore felt in the back of the thigh, leg and foot. The commonest cause is a PROLAPSED INTERVERTEBRAL DISC pressing on a nerve root, but it may also be due to ankylosing SPONDYLITIS and other conditions.

SCLERA the outer layer of the eyeballs which is white and fibrous same at the front of the eye when it becomes the transparent CORNEA.

SCLERITIS inflammation of the white of the eye (SCLERA).

SCLERODERMA a condition in which connective tissue hardens and contracts. The tissue may be the skin, heart, kidney, lung etc. and the condition may be localized or it may spread throughout the body, eventually being fatal. If the skin is affected, it becomes tough and patchily pigmented and may lead to stiff joints and wasting muscles.

SCLEROSIS hardening of tissue, usually after inflammation leading to parts of organs being hard and of no use. It is applied commonly to such changes in the nervous system (MULTIPLE SCLEROSIS); in other organs it is termed FIBROSIS or CIRRHOSIS

SCROTUM the sac that contains the testicles and holds them outside the body, to permit production and storage of sperm at a temperature lower than that of the abdomen.

SEBACEOUS CYST a cyst formed in the duct of a SEBACEOUS GLAND of the skin.

SEBACEOUS GLAND any of the minute glands in the skin that secrete an oily substance called SEBUM. The glands open into hair follicles. Activity of the glands varies with age, puberty being the most active period.

SEBORRHOEA excessive production of SEBUM by the SEBACEOUS GLANDS producing either a build up of dry scurf or oily deposits on the skin. The condition often leads to the development of ACNE.

SEBUM the secretion formed by the SEBACEOUS GLANDS, which forms a thin oily film on the skin, preventing excessive dryness. It also has an antibacterial action.

SECRETION the material produced by a gland.

SEDATIVE a drug that lessens tension and anxiety. Sedatives are hypnotic drugs, e.g. barbiturates, given in doses lower than would bring on sleep.

SEMEN the fluid that contains the sperm which is ejaculated from the penis during copulation.

SENSATION a feeling. The result of stimulation of a sensory receptor producing a nerve impulse which travels on an afferent fibre to the brain.

SENSITIVITY with reference to a SCREENING TEST, the proportion of people with the disease who are identified by the test.

SENSITIZATION a change in the body's response to foreign substances. With the development of an allergy, a person becomes sensitized to a certain ALLERGEN and then becomes hypersensitive. Similarly it may be an acquired reaction when ANTIBODIES develop in response to an ANTIGEN.

SEPSIS the destruction of tissues through putrefaction by bacteria-causing disease, or toxins produced by bacteria.

SEPTAL DEFECT a hole in the SEPTUM or partition between the left and right sides of the heart, whether in the atria (*see* ATRIUM) or VENTRICLES. This condition is a CONGENITAL disorder caused by an abnormal development of the foetal heart. Whether the defect is atrial or ventricular, it allows incorrect circulation of the blood from left to right, from higher pressure to lower. This is called a *shunt*, and results in too much blood flowing through the lungs. PULMONARY HYPERTENSION results and a large shunt may cause heart failure. Surgery can correct the defect, although a small one may not require any treatment.

SEPTIC affected with SEPSIS.

SEPTICAEMIA a term used loosely for any type of blood poisoning. Also a systemic infection with PATHOGENS from an infected part of the body circulating in the bloodstream.

SEPTIC SHOCK a form of shock that occurs due to SEPTICAEMIA. The toxins cause a drastic fall in blood pressure due to tissue damage and blood clotting. Kidneys, heart and lungs are affected and related symptoms include fever, TACHYCAR-DIA or even coma. The condition occurs most in those who already have a serious disease such as cancer, DIABETES, or CIRRHOSIS. Urgent treatment is vital, with antibiotics, oxygen and fluids given intravenously.

SEPTUM a planar dividing feature within a structure of the body; a partition.

SEROUS MEMBRANE a membrane lining a large cavity in the body. The membranes are smooth and transparent and the surfaces are moistened by fluid derived from blood or lymph serum (hence the name). Examples are the PERITONEUM and the PERICARDIUM. Each consists of two layers, the *visceral* which surrounds the organs and the *parietal* which lines the cavity. The two portions are continuous and the surfaces are close together, separated by fluid which permits free movement of the organs.

SERUM a serous fluid. More specifically the clear, sticky fluid that separates from blood and lymph when clotting occurs. In addition to water, serum contains albumin and GLOBULIN with salts, fat, sugar, UREA and other compounds important in disease prevention.

Also, a VACCINE prepared from the serum of a hyperimmune donor for use in protection against a particular infection.

SERUM SICKNESS a hypersensitive reaction that occasionally occurs several days after injection of foreign SERUM, producing rashes, joint pains, fever and swelling of the lymph nodes. It is due to circulating antigen material to which the body responds. It is not a serious condition.

SEX HORMONES steroid hormones responsible for the control of sexual development (primary and SECONDARY SEXUAL CHARACTERISTICS) and reproductive function. The ovaries and testes are the organs primarily involved in hormone production, of which there are three main types: ANDROGENS, the male sex hormones; OESTROGENS and PROGESTERONE, the female sex hormones.

SEXUALLY-TRANSMITTED DISEASES *see* VENEREAL DISEASES.

SHINGLES the common name for herpes zoster (*see* HERPES).

SHOCK acute circulatory failure, when the arterial blood pressure is too low to provide the normal blood supply to the body. The signs are a cold, clammy skin, pallor, CYANOSIS, weak rapid pulse, irregular breathing and dilated pupils. There may also be a reduced flow of urine and confusion or lethargy. There are numerous causes of shock from a reduction in blood volume as after burns, external bleeding, dehydration etc., to reduced heart activity as in CORONARY THROMBOSIS, PULMONARY EMBOLISM, etc.

Certain other circumstances may produce shock, including severe allergic reactions (anaphylactic shock, *see* ANAPHYLAXIS), drugs overdose, emotional shock and so on.

SHORT SIGHT *see* MYOPIA.

SHOULDER BLADE *see* SCAPULA.

SHOULDER GIRDLE *see* PECTORAL GIRDLE.

SIDE-EFFECT the additional and unwanted effect(s) of a drug above the intended action. Sometimes side-effects are harmful and may be stronger than anticipated results of the drug, or something quite different.

SIGMOID COLON the end part of the COLON which is S-shaped.

SILICOSIS a type of PNEUMOCONIOSIS caused by the inhalation of silica as particles of dust. The silica promotes FIBROSIS of the lung tissue resulting in breathlessness and a greater likelihood to contract tuberculosis. Workers in quarrying, mineral mining, sand blasting, etc. are most susceptible.

SINEW the TENDON of a muscle.
SINOATRIAL NODE the natural
heart pacemaker which consists of
specialized muscle cells in the right
atrium. These cells generate
electrical impulses, contract and
initiate contractions in the muscles
of the heart. The AUTONOMIC NERVOUS
SYSTEM supplies the node and certain
hormones also have an effect.
SINUS in general terms a cavity or
channel. Specifically air cavities in
bone as in the bones of the face and
skull. Also a channel, as in the DURA
MATER and which drains venous
blood from the brain.
SINUSITIS inflammation of a SINUS.
It usually refers to the sinuses in the
face which link with the nose and
may there-fore be due to a spread of
infection from the nose. Headaches
and a tenderness over the affected
sinus are typical symptoms with a
pus-containing discharge from the
nose. Persistent infection may
necessitate surgery to drain the
sinus.
SKELETON the rigid, supporting
framework of the body that protects
organs and tissues, provides muscle
attachments, facilitates movement,
and produces red blood cells. There
are 206 bones divided into the axial
skeleton (head and trunk) and the
appendicular skeleton (limbs). The
types of bone are: long (e.g.
humerus), short (e.g. carpals), flat
(parts of the cranium) and irregular
(e.g. the vertebrae).
SKIN the outer layer of the body
comprising an external EPIDERMIS
itself made up of a *stratum corneum*
(horny layer) formed of flat cells that
rub off, being replaced from below.
Beneath this are two more layers
(*stratum lucidum* and *stratum
granulosum*) which act as
intermediate stages between the
stratum corneum and a still lower
layer, the Malpighian layer.
The Malpighian layer is where the

epidermis is produced. The dermis
lies beneath the epidermis and then
follows subcutaneous tissue
composed mainly of fat. The
subcutaneous tissue contains glands
(sweat, SEBACEOUS, etc.), sensory
receptors for pain, pressure and
temperature, nerves, muscles and
blood capillaries.
The skin is a protective layer against
injury and parasites and it moderates
water loss. It is a medium of
temperature control by means of the
sweat glands and blood capillaries
and also the hairs (which provide
insulation).
SKIN GRAFT (*see also* GRAFT) a
piece of skin taken from another site
on the body to cover an injured area,
commonly due to burns. The graft is
normally taken from elsewhere on
the patient's body (*autograft*) but
occasionally from someone else
(*homograft*). A variety of thicknesses
and graft types are used, depending
upon the wound.
SKULL the part of the SKELETON that
forms the head and encloses the
brain. It is made up of 22 bones,
forming the cranium (eight bones)
and fourteen in the face and all
except the mandible are fused along
sutures creating immovable joints.
The mandible (lower jaw) articulates
close to the ears. A large opening at
the base of the skull (FORAMEN
magnum) allows the spinal cord to
pass from the brain to the trunk of
the body.
SLEEP a state of lower awareness
accompanied by reduced metabolic
activity and physical relaxation.
When falling asleep, there is a
change in the brain's electrical
activity. This activity can be
recorded by an ELECTROENCEPHALO-
GRAM (EEG). There are high
amplitude, low frequency waves
(slow-wave sleep) interrupted by
short periods of low amplitude, high
frequency waves. The periods of

high frequency waves are typified by restless sleep with dreams and rapid eye movements, hence the name REM SLEEP, and the EEG is similar to that of a waking person. REM sleep comprises about 25% of the time asleep.

SLING a bandage so arranged as to support an injured limb, usually an arm.

SLIPPED DISC *see* PROLAPSED INTERVERTEBRAL DISC.

SLOUGH dead tissue, usually of limited extent, that after infection separates from the healthy tissue of the rest of the body. In cases of GANGRENE it is possible for limbs to be lost.

SMALL INTESTINE *see* INTESTINE.

SMALLPOX a highly infectious viral disease that has nonetheless been eradicated. Infection results, after about two weeks, in a high fever, head and body aches and vomiting. Eventually red spots appear which change to water and then pus-filled vesicles which on drying out leave scars. The person stays infectious until all scabs are shed. Fever often returns, with DELIRIUM, and although recovery is usual, complications often ensue, e.g. PNEUMONIA. The last naturally-occurring case was in 1977.

SMOOTH MUSCLE *see* INVOLUNTARY MUSCLE.

SOLAR PLEXUS a network of sympathetic nerves and ganglia (*see* GANGLION) behind the stomach, surrounding the coeliac artery. It is a major autonomic PLEXUS of the body where nerves of the sympathetic and parasympathetic nervous system combine (*see individual terms*).

SOMATIC descriptive term meaning relating to the body, as opposed to the mind. More specifically, concerning the *nonreproductive* parts of the body.

SORE a common term for an ulcer or open skin wound.

SOUND an instrument resembling a rod, with a curved end, that is used to explore a body cavity, e.g. the bladder, or to dilate STRICTURES.

SPASM a muscular contraction that is involuntary. Spasms may be part of a more major disorder (e.g. spastic paralysis, convulsions) or they may be specific such as cramp, colic, etc. A heart spasm is known as ANGINA.

SPASTICITY muscular hypertonicity (i.e. an increase in the state of readiness of muscle fibres to contract; an increase in the normal partial contraction) with an increased resistance to stretch. Moderate cases show movement requiring great effort and a lack of normal coordination while slight cases show exaggerated movements that are coordinated.

SPASTIC PARALYSIS weakness of a limb characterized by involuntary muscular contraction and loss of muscular function. As with SPASTICITY it is due to disease of the nerve fibres that usually control movement and reflexes.

SPERMATOZOON (*plural* **SPERMATOZOA**) the mature male reproductive cell, or gamete. It has a head with the HAPLOID nucleus containing half the CHROMOSOME number, and an acrosome (a structure that aids penetration of the egg). Behind the head comes a midpiece with energy-producing MITOCHONDRIA, and then a long tail which propels it forward. A few millilitres of SEMEN is ejaculated during intercourse, containing many millions of spermatozoa.

SPHENOID BONE a bone in the skull that lies behind the eyes.

SPHINCTER a circular muscle around an opening. The opening is closed totally or partially by contraction of the muscle, e.g. the anal sphincter around the anus.

SPINAL COLUMN (SPINE,

BACKBONE, VERTEBRAL COLUMN) the bony and slightly flexible column that forms a vital part of the SKELETON. It encloses the SPINAL CORD, articulates with other bones, e.g. the skull and ribs, and provides attachments for muscles. It consists of bones, the vertebrae, between which are discs of fibrocartilage (the intervertebral discs). From the top, the column comprises 7 cervical, 12 thoracic, 5 lumbar, 5 sacral and 4 coccygeal vertebrae. In adults the last two groups are fused to from the sacrum and coccyx, respectively.

SPINAL CORD the part of the CENTRAL NERVOUS SYSTEM that runs from the brain, through the SPINAL COLUMN. Both GREY and WHITE MATTER are present, the former as an H-shaped core within the latter. A hollow core in the grey matter forms the central canal which contains the cerebrospinal fluid. The cord is covered by MENINGES and it contains both sensory and motor NEURONS. Thirty-one pairs of spinal nerves arise from the cord, passing out between the arches of the vertebrae.

SPLEEN a roughly ovoid organ, coloured a deep purple, which is situated on the left of the body, behind and below the stomach. It is surrounded by a peritoneal membrane and contains a mass of lymphoid tissue. MACROPHAGES in the spleen destroy microorganisms by PHAGOCYTOSIS.

The spleen produces lymphocytes, leucocytes, plasma cells and blood platelets (see individual entries). It also stores red blood cells for use in emergencies. Release of red blood cells is facilitated by SMOOTH MUSCLE under the control of the SYMPATHETIC NERVOUS SYSTEM, and when this occurs, the familiar pain called *stitch* may be experienced. The spleen removes worn out red blood cells, conserving the iron for further production in the bone marrow. Although the spleen performs many functions, it can be removed without detriment and as a result there is an increase in size of the lymphatic glands.

SPLINT a support that holds a broken bone in the correct and stable position until healing is complete.

SPRAIN an injury to ligaments (or muscles, or tendons) around a joint, caused by a sudden overstretching. Pain and swelling may occur and treatment comprises, in the main, avoiding use of the affected joint.

SPUTUM saliva and mucus from the respiratory tract.

SQUINT (or STRABISMUS) an abnormal condition in which the eyes are crossed. There are two types, paralytic and non-paralytic. The paralytic type is due to a muscular or neurological malfunction, while a non-paralytic squint is caused by a defect in the actual relative position of the eyes. Some squints can be corrected by surgery.

STENOSIS the abnormal narrowing of a blood vessel, heart valve or similar structure.

STERNUM the breastbone.

STEROID one of a group of compounds resembling cholesterol, that are made up of four carbon rings fused together. The group includes the sterols (e.g. cholesterol), BILE acids, some HORMONES, and vitamin D. Synthetic versions act like steroid hormones and include derivatives of the glucocorticoids used as anti-inflammatory agents for RHEUMATOID ARTHRITIS; oral contraceptives, usually OESTROGEN and PROGESTERONE derivatives; anabolic steroids such as testosterone used to treat OSTEOPOROSIS and wasting.

STERTOR noisy breathing, similar to snoring, often heard in patients who are deeply unconscious.

STIFFNESS a condition with numerous causes, that results in a reduced movement in joints and muscles. The cause may be quite straightforward, e.g. physical injury, or it may be due to disease such as RHEUMATISM, MENINGITIS or central nervous system diseases.

STILLBIRTH the birth of any child that provides no evidence of life.

STIMULANT any drug or other agent that increases the rate of activity of an organ or system within the body. This assumes that the target organ is capable of increased activity which merely requires the necessary stimulus.

STITCH a sharp pain in the side often due to cramp after hard exertion (*see also* SPLEEN).

STOMA (*plural* STOMATA) an opening made in the abdominal surface to accommodate a tube from the colon or ileum. This operation is undertaken because of malignancy or inflammatory bowel diseases, e.g. Crohn's disease.

STOMACH an expansion of the alimentary canal that lies between the OESOPHAGUS and the DUODENUM. It has thick walls of SMOOTH MUSCLE that contract to manipulate the food, and its exits are controlled by SPHINCTERS, the cardiac anteriorly and the pyloric at the junction with the duodenum (*see* PYLORUS). Mucosal cells in the lining secrete GASTRIC JUICE. The food is reduced to an acidic semi-liquid which is moved on to the duodenum.

STOOLS *see* FAECES.

STRANGULATION the constriction or closure of a passage or vessel. This may be due to the intestine twisting, or herniation of the intestine. Strangulation of a blood vessel and/or airway affects the organs being supplied and if these are vital organs are affected, can prove fatal.

STRAPPING the application of layers of adhesive plaster to cover part of the body and maintain moderate pressure, so as to prevent too much movement and provide rest, as with fractured ribs.

STREPTOCOCCUS a genus of Gram-positive (*see* GRAM'S STAIN) spherical bacteria that form chains. Many species are responsible for a variety of infections including scarlet fever, ENDOCARDITIS and pneumonia.

STRESS FRACTURE a fracture created by making excessive demands on the body, as commonly happens in sport. Treatment involves rest and analgesics for the pain.

STRICTURE a narrowing of a passage in the body, e.g. the URETHRA, OESOPHAGUS, or URETER. It may result from inflammation, a spasm, growth of a tumour or pressure from surrounding organs. In many cases it is due to ulceration and contraction of the subsequent scar tissue. With a urethral stricture, it becomes increasingly difficult to pass urine.

STRIDOR the noise created on breathing in when there is a narrowing of the upper airway, especially the LARYNX.

STROKE (*or* CEREBRO-VASCULAR ACCIDENT) the physical effects, involving some form of paralysis, that result from an interruption to the brain's blood supply. The effect in the brain is secondary and the cause lies in the heart or blood vessels and may be a THROMBOSIS, EMBOLUS, or HAEMOR-RHAGE. The severity of a stroke varies greatly from a temporary weakness in a limb, or tingling, to paralysis, coma and death.

STYE a bacterial infection and inflammation of a gland at the base of an eyelash, resulting in a pus-filled cyst.

SUBARACHNOID HAEMOR-RHAGE bleeding into the SUBARACHNOID SPACE due often to a ruptured cerebral ANEURYSM. Initial symptoms are a severe headache, stiff neck, followed by vomiting, drowsiness and there may be a brief period of unconsciousness after the event. Brain damage is possible but severe haemorrhages may result in death.

SUBARACHNOID SPACE the space between the arachnid and pia mater MENINGES covering the brain and spinal cord. It contains cerebrospinal fluid and blood vessels.

SUBCUTANEOUS general term meaning beneath the skin.

SUBDURAL term meaning below the dura mater, and referring to the space between this and the arachnoid MENINGES around the brain.

SUBPHRENIC ABSCESS an abscess occurring beneath the diaphragm and commonly on the right side. It may be due to infection after an operation or perforation of an organ, e.g. a peptic ulcer. Surgery is usually necessary although antibiotics may be effective.

SUDDEN INFANT DEATH SYNDROME (*or* COT DEATH) the sudden death of a baby, often occurring overnight, from unknown causes. A significant proportion (c. 20% in U.K.) of infant deaths occur this way. Although the cause is unknown numerous suggestions have been put forward from viral infection and allergic reaction to poor breathing control that be particularly susceptible to mild infections. Research continues.

SUNBURN skin damage caused by exposure to the ultra-violet rays in sunlight. This may vary from a reddening of the skin and itching to formation of blisters which can cause shock if a large area is affected. Fair-skinned people are more susceptible than others and it is advisable to take sun in gradual stages.

SUNSTROKE *see* HEATSTROKE.
SUPINE the position in which

someone is lying on their back, face upwards.

SUPPURATION pus formation, whether on the surface (ulceration) or more deep seated (as with an ABSCESS).

SUTURE the means whereby a wound or incision is closed in surgery, using threads of silk or catgut. There are several types of suture to deal with diverse situations. Also, a type of joint across which there is no movement, e.g. as in the skull, where there are several sutures.

SWAB a general term applied to a pad of material used in various ways. It can be used to clean wounds, apply medication, remove blood during operations, and obtain samples from infected areas, e.g. throat, for further examination.

SWEAT *see* PERSPIRATION.

SWEAT GLANDS the glands in the EPIDERMIS of SKIN that project into the dermis and are under the control of the sympathetic nervous system (*see also* PERSPIRATION). The glands occur over most of the body but are especially abundant on the forehead, palms of the hands and soles of the feet and under the arms.

SYMPATHETIC the term for a symptom or disease that occurs as a result of disease elsewhere in the body, e.g. injury of one eye and a related inflammation in the other due to them being connected by the lymphatics.

SYMPATHETIC NERVOUS SYSTEM with the parasympathetic nervous system (and acting in opposition to it), this makes up the AUTONOMIC NERVOUS SYSTEM. NORADRENALINE and ADRENALINE are the main NEUROTRANSMITTERS released by its nerve endings. Its functions include raising the heart beat rate, constricting blood vessels and inhibiting secretion of saliva.

SYMPTOM any evidence of a disease or disorder.

SYNAPSE the junction between two nerve cells, at which there is a minute gap. A nerve impulse bridges the gap via a NEUROTRANSMITTER. The chemical diffuses across the gap that connects the axon of one nerve cell to the dendrites of the next. Some brain cells have many thousand synapses.

SYNCOPE (*or* FAINTING) a temporary loss of consciousness due to a fall in blood pressure and a reduced supply of blood to the brain. It may occur after standing for a long time (particularly in hot weather), after shock or injury. Typical signs which occur before an attack are sweating and a feeling of light-headedness.

SYNDROME a number of symptoms and signs that in combination together constitute a particular condition.

SYNOVIAL MEMBRANE (*or* SYNOVIUM) the inner membrane of a capsule that encloses a joint that moves freely. It secretes into the joint a thick lubricating fluid (synovial fluid) which may build up after injury to cause pain.

SYNOVITIS inflammation of the SYNOVIAL MEMBRANE that lines a joint capsule. The result is swelling with pain. It is associated with rheumatic disease, injury or infection (e.g. chronic tuberculosis). The treatment depends upon the cause of the condition and often a sample of the synovial fluid is taken for examination.

SYRINGE an instrument used for injecting fluids into the body or the removal of body fluids for examination. In such cases, it comprises a hollow needle connected to a piston within a tube. Larger metal syringes are used to wash the outer ear and remove wax.

SYSTEMIC general term referring to the body as a whole.

SYSTOLE the contraction of the heart that alternates with the resting phase (diastole). It usually refers to ventricular systole which at 0.3 seconds is three times longer than atrial systole.

SYSTOLIC PRESSURE *see* BLOOD PRESSURE.

T

TACHYCARDIA increased rate of heart beat which may be caused naturally as with exercise or be symptomatic of disease.

TALUS the ankle bone which articulates with the lower leg bones (TIBIA and FIBULA) above and also with the heel bone (*calcaneus*) below (*see* TARSUS).

TARGET CELL an abnormal form of ERYTHROCYTE (red blood cell) which is large and has a ringed appearance when stained and viewed microscopically, resembling a target. These cells are present in several kinds of anaemia including those due to iron-deficiency.

TARSUS a part of the foot in the region of the instep consisting of seven bones, chiefly the TALUS and the *calcaneus* (heel bone) and also the cuboid, navicular and three cuneiform bones.

TASTE BUDS the sensory receptors responsible for the perception of taste, located in the grooves around the papillae of the TONGUE, in the epiglottis, parts of the PHARYNX and soft palate. The taste buds are stimulated by the presence of dissolved food in the saliva and messages are sent via nerves to the brain where the information is interpreted and perceived.

TAXIS the returning to their normal position of displaced organs, parts of organs or bones by manipulation (*see* HERNIA).

TEETH *see* TOOTH.

TEMPERATURE (of the body) the normal body temperature is around 37°C (98.4°F) but it varies considerably both between individuals and in one person throughout the day. In addition, temperature differences occur between various areas of the body being lower in the skin than internally.

TEMPLE the side of the head above the level of the eye and the ear.

TEMPORAL relating or referring to the temple, e.g. *temporal artery*.

TEMPORAL LOBE one of the main areas of the CEREBRAL CORTEX in each of the CEREBRAL HEMISPHERES of the brain, occurring in the TEMPORAL region of the skull. A cleft known as the *lateral sulcus* separates it from the frontal lobe.

TEMPORAL LOBE EPILEPSY EPILEPSY which is centred within the temporal lobe caused by disease within the cortex. It is characterized by hallucinations involving the senses of taste, smell, hearing and sight and memory disturbances. During an attack, the person usually remains conscious but not fully and normally aware, and afterwards may not have any memory of what has occurred.

TENDINITIS inflammation of a tendon which often results from excessive or unaccustomed exercise but may also result from infection. Treatment involves rest, possibly splinting of an affected joint and corticosteroid injections, and the taking of ANALGESIC drugs.

TENDON a tough and inelastic white cord composed of bundles of COLLAGEN fibres which attaches a muscle to a bone.A tendon concentrates the pull of the muscle onto one point on the bone and the length and thickness varies considerably. The fibres of a tendon pass into, and become continuous with, those of the bone it serves.

Many tendons are enclosed in tendon sheaths lined with SYNOVIAL MEMBRANE containing synovial fluid which reduces friction and enables easy movement to occur.

TENNIS ELBOW a form of TENDINITIS affecting the tendon at the outer part of the elbow which becomes inflamed and painful. It is caused by hard and excessive use of the arm and the treatment involves rest and corticosteroid injections.

TESTICLE (TESTIS) one of the pair of male sex organs which are situated within the SCROTUM and which produce spermatozoa and secrete the hormone TESTOSTERONE. The testicles develop within the abdomen of the foetus but descend around the time of birth into the scrotum.

TESTIS *see* TESTICLE.

TESTOSTERONE the male sex hormone secreted by the TESTES (*see also* ANDROGEN).

TETANUS a very serious and sometimes fatal infectious disease, the non-medical name for which is *lockjaw*. It is caused by the bacterium *Clostridium tetani*, spores of which enter through a wound. Rapid multiplication of the bacteria produces a toxin which affects the nerves resulting in rigidity and spasm of muscles. Often there is high fever and the spasms cause extreme agony. If respiratory muscles are involved death may occur by asphyxia. Effective antitoxin is available, although its effects are not permanent and it needs to be regularly maintained. Antibiotics such as penicillin are also effective against the bacteria.

THALAMUS one of a pair of masses of grey matter located within each side of the forebrain. Each is a centre for co-ordinating and relaying the sensory information concerned with all the senses apart from that of smell.

THIGH the part of the leg above the knee.

THORAX the chest.

THROMBIN an enzyme derived from prothrombin, its inactive precursor, which is formed and is active during the final stages of blood clotting (*see* COAGULATION).

THROMBOEMBOLISM the situation in which a blood clot (THROMBUS) forms in one part of the circulation, usually a vein in the leg (phlebothrombosis), and a portion breaks off and becomes lodged elsewhere causing a total blockage (EMBOLISM). The embolism often involves the pulmonary artery or one of its branches and this is known as PULMONARY EMBOLISM.

THROMBOPHLEBITIS inflammation of the wall of a vein along with clot formation in the affected section of the vessel. This is a complication of pregnancy and may be dangerous, involving a deep vein thrombosis which can result in PULMONARY EMBOLISM. The condition known as white leg, (plegmasia alba dolens) is thrombophlebitis especially of the femoral vein which can occur after childbirth.

THROMBOSIS the process of clotting within a blood vessel producing a THROMBUS. It may occur within an artery or vein, often one which is diseased or damaged, and can be very serious or even fatal, e.g. STROKE, CORONARY THROMBOSIS.

THROMBUS a blood clot within a vessel which partially or totally obstructs the circulation.

THYMUS a gland, divided into two lobes, which is present in the neck and which forms a vital part of the immune system. It is especially large in children and important in the development of the immune response and the production of lymphoid tissue. After puberty, the thymus gradually begins to shrink.

Bone marrow cells, known as *stem cells*, undergo maturation within the thymus and one group, the *T. lymphocytes*, are dependent upon the gland. These are very important cells in the body which produce ANTIBODIES.

THYROID GLAND a bilobed endocrine gland situated at the base and front of the neck. It is enclosed by fibrous tissue and well-supplied with blood, and internally consists of numerous vesicles containing a jelly-like colloidal substance. These vesicles produce thyroid hormone, which is rich in iodine, under the control of *thyroid stimulating hormone* (THYROTROPHIN STIMULATING HORMONE) released from the PITUITARY GLAND. Two hormones are produced by the gland, thyroxine and triiodothyronine, which are essential for the regulation of metabolism and growth. *See also* MYXOEDEMA and HYPERTHYROIDISM.

THYROXINE an important hormone produced by the thyroid gland and used medically to treat conditions resulting from underactivity of this gland, e.g. cretinism and MYXOEDEMA.

TIBIA the larger of the two bones in the lower leg known as the shin bone articulating above with the FEMUR and with the TALUS of the ankle below.

TINNITUS any ringing or buzzing sound in the ear which does not have a real external cause. Many disorders of the ear can cause this, for example, hardened wax, Ménière's disease, drugs including aspirin and quinine, and damage to the auditory nerve. In many cases no underlying cause is found.

TONGUE the muscular and highly mobile organ attached to the floor of the mouth, the three main functions of which are manipulation of food during chewing prior to swallowing, taste and production of speech. The three areas of the tongue are the tip, body and root and it is covered with a mucous membrane which unites with that of the mouth and pharynx. The tongue is anchored at the root by various muscles which attach it to the back of the mouth. In addition, the undersurface of the tongue is attached in the midline to the floor of the mouth by a fold of mucous membrane called the *frenulum lingae*. The tongue has a furred appearance because its surface is covered with minute projections called papillae, of which there are three different kinds, filiform, fungiform and circumvallate. There are grooves surrounding the papillae in which the TASTE BUDS occur. The tongue is well supplied with blood and receives branches from five different nerves on each side.

TONSILLITIS inflammation of the tonsils caused by bacterial or viral infection. The symptoms include a severe sore throat causing painful swallowing, accompanied by fever and earache, especially in children. The tonsils are swollen and white in appearance due to infected material exuded from them and glands in the neck are enlarged.

TONSILS usually refers to the two small masses of lymphoid tissue situated on either side at the back of the mouth (the *palatine tonsils*). However, another pair occur below the tongue which are the *lingual tonsils* while the ADENOIDS are the PHARYNGEAL TONSILS. All are part of the body's protective mechanism against infection.

TOOTH a hard structure used for biting and chewing. Each tooth consists of a *root* embedded in a socket within the jawbone to which it is attached by the fibrous *periodontal membrane*. The projecting part of the tooth is called the *crown* which is covered with a hard resistant layer of *enamel*,

(composed primarily of calcium phosphate and calcium carbonate). The root is covered with a thin hard layer of cementum.
Most of the interior of the tooth consists of *dentine*, a hard ivory-like substance which surrounds the inner core or pulp. The pulp contains blood vessels and nerve fibres and is connected with the dentine by means of fine cellular processes. There are four different types of teeth, canine, incisor, premolar and molar.

TORSION twisting, often referring to an abnormal state of the whole or part of an organ which impairs the nerve and blood supply. Examples are a torsion of a loop of bowel or of the spermatic cord of the testicle. Surgery is usually required to correct a torsion.

TOUCH the sense which is conferred by specialized sensory receptors present in the skin (and also in muscles and other areas of the body), which enable sensations of pain, temperature, pressure and touch to be perceived. The sense organs involved are specially adapted to respond to particular sensations conveying their messages to the brain along different nerve pathways.

TOURNIQUET a device used to arrest bleeding, usually from an artery in a limb, which may be a length of bandage, rubber tube or cord tied tightly round generally as an emergency measure. Direct pressure on a wound is now considered to be preferable as a first aid measure, because a tourniquet can deprive all the tissues of oxygen by arresting the circulation, and there is a risk of damage and of gangrene.

TOXAEMIA blood poisoning resulting from the toxins produced by rapidly multiplying bacteria at a localized site of infection such as an abscess. Symptoms are varied including fever, vomiting and diarrhoea and a general feeling of being unwell. The source of the infection has to be treated with antibiotic drugs. Toxaemia of pregnancy involves two relatively rare conditions known as ECLAMPSIA and PRE-ECLAMPSIA.

TOXIC SHOCK SYNDROME a state of acute shock due to SEPTICAEMIA and caused by toxins produced by *staphylococcal* bacteria. The symptoms include high fever, skin rash and diarrhoea and can prove rapidly fatal if not adequately treated with antibiotics, especially penicillin and *cephalosporin*, along with fluid and salt replacement. The syndrome is associated with the use of tampons by women during menstruation but can also occur in other people, and is in all cases rare.

TOXIN a poison produced by bacteria and by many species of plant and also present in snake venom. In the body, a toxin acts as an ANTIGEN and provokes the production of special antibodies called antitoxins. The antitoxins produced may be used in IMMUNIZA-TION to protect against the disease as with tetanus and diphtheria. An *endotoxin* is contained within the bacterial cell and only released when the organism dies and decays. Endotoxins do not provoke antitoxin production (*see* TOXOID).

TOXOPLASMOSIS an infectious disease caused by a protozoan organism known as *Toxoplasma*. The infection is either transmitted by eating undercooked meat or through direct contact with contaminated soil or especially with infected cats. This form of the infection is mild and causes few ill effects. However, a much more serious form of the disease can be passed from a mother infected during pregnancy to her unborn baby. The newborn infant may suffer from HYDROCEPHALUS,

mental retardation, blindness or may even be stillborn. Treatment is by means of sulphonamide drugs and pyrimethamine.

TRACHEA the windpipe which is the part of the air passage that is situated between the LARYNX and the bronchi.

TRACHEOSTOMY (*or* **TRACHE-OTOMY**) a surgical procedure in which a hole is made in the trachea to allow direct access of air to the lower respiratory passages. This may be performed in an emergency if there is an obstruction in breathing. However, usually this operation is carried out in hospital, especially on patients in intensive therapy who require long-term artificial ventilation.

TRANSFUSION *see* BLOOD TRANSFUSION.

TRANSPLANTATION the transfer of an organ or tissue from one person to another (*allotransplant*) or within the body of an individual (*autotransplant*), i.e., skin and bone grafting. The person from whom the organ is obtained is known as the *donor* and the one who receives it is known as the *recipient*.
Organ transplants involving the kidney, heart, bone marrow, cornea, lungs and liver have all become more common. Success varies but is improving in all areas especially with the advent of *immunosuppressive* drugs to prevent organ rejection by the recipient's immune system. *See also* IMMUNOSUPPRESSION and GRAFT.

TRAUMA an event which causes physical damage such as a fracture or an emotional shock brought about by a harmful and upsetting circumstance.

TREMOR involuntary movements which may involve the whole of a muscle or only part of it and produce fine trembling or more pronounced shaking. Tremors are classified according to the type of movement produced and are a symptom of many diseases including CHOREA, MULTIPLE SCLEROSIS and PARKINSONISM.

TRICEPS a three-headed muscle present in the upper arm which extends the forearm.

TRICUSPID VALVE a valve with three flaps or cusps that controls the passage of blood from the right ATRIUM to the right VENTRICLE of the heart and normally prevents backflow (*see* HEART).

TRIGEMINAL NERVE the fifth and largest of the cranial nerves which has three divisions, the *mandibular, maxillary* and *ophthalmic* nerves. The ophthalmic and maxillary are sensory nerves and the mandibular has both sensory and motor functions. Hence the trigeminal nerve is involved in the relaying and perception of sensations (temperature, touch, pain, etc.) from the whole of the face and mouth and also in controlling the muscles involved in chewing.

TUBERCULOSIS a group of infections caused by the bacillus (bacterium) *Mycobacterium tuberculosis* of which pulmonary tuberculosis of the lungs (consumption or phthisis) is the best known form. The pulmonary disease is acquired through inhalation of air containing the organism from an infected person, or dust laden with bacteria.

If the infection is severe, symptoms include fever, wasting, night sweats and the coughing up of blood. The bacteria may enter the blood stream and spread throughout the body setting up numerous tubercles in other tissues (*miliary tuberculosis*). The organism may also be acquired by eating contaminated food, especially milk, in which case the production of a primary complex in abdominal lymph nodes can lead to PERITONITIS. Tuberculosis affects people throughout the world (about 6000 new cases each year in England

and Wales). Many people acquire the infection and recover without suspecting its presence and the disease is curable with antibiotics, e.g. streptomycin. In addition, BCG VACCINATION as a preventive measure is given to children in the UK, in addition to X-ray screening to detect carriers.

TUMOUR any abnormal swelling occurring in any part of the body consisting of an unusual growth of tissue and which may be malignant or benign. Tumours tend to be classified according to the tissue of which they are composed, e.g. FIBROMA (mainly fibrous tissue) and myoma (largely muscle fibres).

TURGOR a state of being distended, engorged or swollen.

TYMPANIC MEMBRANE the eardrum which separates the middle and outer ears and which vibrates in response to sound waves transmitting the vibrations to one of the ear ossicles (the *malleus*). *See* EAR.

TYPHOID FEVER a severe infectious disease of the digestive system which is caused by the bacterium *Salmonella typhi* and causes symptoms including a rise in temperature, a rash on the abdomen and chest, headache and nosebleeds. The temperature rise occurs in a characteristic fashion known as a *step-ladder temperature*. In severe cases there may be ulceration of the intestinal wall leading to PERITONITIS if an ulcer bursts, or haemorrhage from the bowels and inflammation of the lungs, SPLEEN and bones. In these cases the disease can prove to be fatal. The infection is acquired through ingesting contaminated food or water hence preventive measures involving high standards of hygiene and sanitation are important. Drug treatment is by means of antibiotics such as chloramphenicol and ampicillin. Inoculation with TAB vaccine confers temporary immunity.

ULCER

U

ULCER a break on the skin surface
or on the MUCOUS MEMBRANE lining
within the body cavities that may be
inflamed and fails to heal. Ulcers of
the skin include bedsores and
varicose ulcers (which are caused by
defective circulation). For ulcers of
the alimentary tract, see DUODENAL
ULCER, GASTRIC ULCER and PEPTIC
ULCER.

ULNA one of the two bones making
up the forearm. It is the inner and
longer of the two bones (the other
being the radius). It articulates with
the radius at both ends and
additionally with the humerus above,
and indirectly with the wrist below.

UMBILICAL CORD the cord
connecting the foetus to the placenta,
containing two arteries and one vein.
It is approximately 60cm long and
after birth it is severed and the stump
shrivels to leave a scar, the navel or
umbilicus.

UMBILICUS the navel (*see
UMBILICAL CORD*).

UNCONSCIOUSNESS the state of
being partially or totally unaware of
the surroundings and lacking in
response to stimuli. Sleep is a
natural form of unconsciousness.
Unnatural states of unconsciousness
can be due to numerous causes
including injuries to the brain
resulting in compression or
concussion, fainting due to
insufficient blood supply to the
brain, EPILEPSY, poisoning and
various diseases, e.g. DIABETES
MELLITUS.

UNGUAL a term meaning relating
to the fingernails or toenails.

UNGUIS a fingernail or toenail.

URAEMIA the condition where
there is excess UREA in the blood due
to kidney disease or failure. Waste
products are usually excreted by the

kidneys but accumulation in the
blood leads to headaches, drowsiness
and lethargy, nausea and vomiting
and diarrhoea. Eventually, without
treatment, death follows. Haemodial-
ysis on a kidney machine may be
necessary or even a renal transplant.

UREA a metabolic byproduct of the
chemical breakdown of protein and
the form in which excess nitrogen is
removed from the body, in urine. It
is formed in the LIVER and taken in
the blood to the KIDNEYS. The amount
excreted daily is 30-35gm.

URETER the tubes joining the
KIDNEYS to the bladder and through
which urine passes. The muscular
ureter walls contract to force urine
into the bladder.

URETHRA the duct carrying urine
from the bladder out of the body. It
is about 3.5cm long in women and
20cm in men. The male urethra runs
through the penis and also forms the
ejaculatory duct.

URETHRITIS inflammation of the
mucous lining of the urethra which
may be associated with cystitis,
often being the cause of the latter.
The commonest cause or urethritis is
gonorrhoea (*specific*). Alternatively,
it may be due to infection with
microorganisms (causing *non-
specific* urethritis). The symptoms
include pain on passing urine, a
discharge, and possible inflamma-
tions in other organs such as the
bladder and testicle.

URINARY ORGANS the system
responsible for the extraction of
components from the blood to form
urine, its storage and periodic
discharge from the body. The organs
are the kidneys, ureters, bladder and
urethra (*see individual entries*).

URINARY TRACT the system of
ducts that permit movement of urine
out of the body from the kidneys, i.e.
the URETERS, BLADDER and URETHRA.

URINATION (*or* **MICTURITION**)
the discharge of urine from the body

via the URETHRA. It is begun by a voluntary relaxation of the sphincter muscle below the bladder.

URINE the body's fluid waste excreted by the KIDNEYS. The waste products include UREA, URIC ACID and creatinine (produced by muscles) with salt, phosphates and sulphates and ammonia also present. In a solution with about 95-96% water, there may be 100 or more compounds but the vast majority occur only in trace amounts. Many diseases alter the quantity and composition of urine and its analysis is standard procedure to assist diagnosis of diseases.

URINE RETENTION the condition when urine is produced by the kidneys but it is retained in the bladder. This may be due to an obstruction, or a weakness in the bladder (less common). Enlargement of the PROSTATE GLAND is a common cause of blockage. It may also be caused by a STRICTURE due to injury scar or ulceration.

URTICARIA (*or* **NETTLE RASH**) an allergic reaction by an individual to some substance to which they are hypersensitive, in which the allergic response is manifested on the skin. Raised red patches develop which may last for hours or days. There is intense itching. The sensitivity may be to certain foods, e.g. shellfish, and the effect may occur anywhere on the body, but commonly erupts on the face and trunk. If it also affects the tongue or throat, there is danger of a blockage of the airway which would need urgent attention.

UTERINE relating to the UTERUS.

UTERUS (*or* **WOMB**) a vaguely pear-shaped organ within the cavity of the pelvis that is specialized for the growth and nourishment of a foetus. During pregnancy it enlarges considerably and the SMOOTH MUSCLE walls thicken. Contractions of the muscular wall push the foetus out

via the vagina at childbirth. If there is no pregnancy the lining undergoes periodic changes (MENSTRUATION).

UVEA the middle pigmented layer of the EYE consisting of the IRIS, choroid and ciliary body.

VACCINATION the production of immunity to a disease by inoculation with a VACCINE or a specially prepared material that stimulates the production of antibodies. It was used initially to refer only to cowpox virus (which also protected against SMALLPOX) but now is synonymous with inoculation, in immunizing against disease.

VACCINE a modified preparation of a BACTERIUM or VIRUS that is no longer dangerous but will stimulate development of antibodies and therefore confer immunity against actual infection with the disease. Other vaccines consist of specific toxins (e.g. tetanus), or dead bacteria (e.g. cholera and typhoid). Live but weakened organisms are used against smallpox and tuberculosis.

VAGINA the lower part of the female reproductive tract that leads from the uterus to the outside. It receives the erect penis during sexual intercourse, the semen being ejaculated into the upper part from where the sperms pass through the CERVIX and UTERUS to the FALLOPIAN TUBES. The vagina is essentially a muscular tube lined with mucous membrane.

VAGUS the tenth cranial nerve which comprises motor, sensory, vasodilator and secretory fibres. It supplies the muscles for swallowing and fibres go to the heart, throat, lungs and stomach and other organs in the abdomen. It also carries the taste sensation from the mouth.

VALVE a structure within an organ or vessel that restricts flow to one direction, whether the fluid be blood or lymph. The valves comprise cusps on the vessel wall. The cusp is like a membranous pocket that fills with blood should it flow back and the cusps distend and close the valve.

VALVULAR HEART DISEASE affects mainly the AORTIC and MITRAL VALVES which may narrow (STENOSIS) or weaken. Aortic valve disease is associated more with old age while mitral valve disease is rheumatic in origin.

VALVULITIS inflammation of a valve, particularly in the heart. It is commonly due to rheumatic fever.

VAPORIZER a device that produces a mist of liquid medication for inhalation. It is commonly used in the treatment of asthma.

VARICOSE VEINS veins that have become stretched, distended and twisted. The superficial veins in the legs are often affected although it may occur elsewhere. Causes include congenitally defective valves, obesity, pregnancy and thrombophlebitis (inflammation of the wall of a vein with secondary THROMBOSIS in the affected part of the vein). Elastic support is a common treatment although alternatives are SCLEROTHERAPY and PHLEBECTOMY.

VAS a vessel or duct, especially those carrying blood, lymph or spermatozoa.

VASCULAR relating to blood vessels; supplied with blood vessels.

VASCULITIS inflammation of the blood vessels that may cause damage to the linings and cause narrowing. It may result from several conditions including acute NEPHRITIS and SERUM SICKNESS.

VAS DEFERENS the tubes that join the testes to the ejaculatory duct via the PROSTATE GLAND. It carries spermatozoa to the URETHRA on

ejaculation, aided by contraction of its muscular wall.

VASOCONSTRICTION the narrowing of blood vessels with a consequent reduction in blood supply to that part of the body supplied. A variety of circumstances can cause vasoconstriction including cold and shock.

VASODILATION (VASODILATA-TION) the increase in diameter of blood vessels producing a lowering of blood pressure.

VASOPRESSIN (ANTIDIURETIC HORMONE) a PITUITARY GLAND hormone that constricts blood vessels and reduces urine secretion by increasing the quantity of water reabsorbed by the KIDNEY.

VASOVAGAL ATTACK fainting, precipitated by a slowing of the heart and a fall in blood pressure. This may be due to shock, severe pain, fear, etc. and is caused by excessive stimulation of the VAGUS nerve which participates in the control of breathing and the circulation.

VECTOR commonly an insect that carries parasitic microorganisms between people, or from animals to people, e.g. mosquitoes carrying malaria.

VEIN one of the numerous blood vessels carrying deoxygenated blood to the right atrium of the heart (the one exception is the PULMONARY vein). Each vein has three tissue layers, similar to the layers of the heart. Veins are less elastic than arteries and collapse when cut. They also contain VALVES to prevent backflow.

VENA CAVA either of two major veins carrying blood from other veins to the right ATRIUM of the heart. The *inferior* vena cava takes blood from the body below the DIAPHRAGM and the *superior* vena cava takes blood from the head, neck, arms and thorax.

VENEREAL DISEASE (*or*** SEXUALLY TRANSMITTED**

DISEASE) a disease transmitted by sexual intercourse. This includes AIDS, syphilis, gonorrhoea, non-specific urethritis, etc.

VENOM the poisonous substance produced by snakes, scorpions, etc. which in humans may produce only localized pain and swelling, or in serious cases cause more general effects and even death.

VENTILATION the means whereby air passes into and out of the lungs, aided by movement of the diaphragm. *Artificial* ventilation is the usse of a machine (VENTILATOR) to regulate and perform a person's breathing. This may be during an operation. Also, damage to the relevant part of the brain, chest injury, lung disease or nerve and muscle disorders may all require the use of artificial ventilation.

VENTILATOR the machine used to provide an air supply to the lungs of patients who cannot breathe normally for themselves. Blood gases and other body functions can be monitored at the same time.

VENTRICLE one of the two major chambers within the heart. They are thick-walled and muscular and form the main pumping chamber. The right ventricle receives blood from the right ATRIUM and venae cavae and its outflow is the pulmonary artery. The left ventricle takes blood from the pulmonary vein via the left atrium, and its outflow is the AORTA. Also cavities within the brain, filled with cerebrospinal fluid.

VENTRICULAR FIBRILLATION a rapid ARRHYTHMIA of the ventricle which is dangerous.

VERRUCA a term for WART.

VERTEBRA *(plural* VERTE-BRAE) any of the bones making up the vertebral column. Each has a cavity (the vertebral canal or foramen) and various processes for attachment of muscles or articulation of adjacent vertebrae. The spinal

cord passes through the vertebral canal (*see* SPINAL COLUMN).

VERTIGO a condition in which a person has a false sensation of imbalance and of the surroundings moving. It is commonly a sensation of spinning but may be as if the ground is tilting. The semicircular canals of the ear are fundamental in the maintenance of balance and vertigo is generally due to some problem with this mechanism or with the appropriate centres in the brain.

VESICULAR BREATHING soft, normal sounds of breathing heard in the lung by means of a stethoscope. The sounds change when the lungs are diseased and the different sounds help a doctor diagnose the disease.

VESSEL any tube that carries fluid, particularly blood or lymph.

VILLUS (*plural* VILLI) *see* JEJUNUM.

VIRAL HAEMORRHAGIC FEVER a viral disease with a high mortality rate. After the incubation period there is headache, fever, severe internal bleeding, diarrhoea and vomiting. Death may follow, usually eight or nine days later. Serum taken from someone recovering from the disease is a useful source of antibodies.

VIRAL PNEUMONIA an acute lung infection caused by one of a number of viruses. The symptoms include fever, headache, muscle pains and a thick sputum associated with the cough. It often ocurs after a viral infection and treatment, in the main, deals with the symptoms only.

VIRULENCE the ability of a bacterium of virus to cause disease, measured by numbers of people infected, the speed with which it spreads through the body, etc.

VIRUS the smallest microbe that is completely parasitic, because it is only capable of replication within the cells of its host. Viruses infect animals, plants and microorganisms. Viruses are classified according to

VISCERA

186

their nucleic acids and can contain double or single-stranded DNA or RNA. In an infection the virus binds to the host cells and then penetrates to release the viral DNA or RNA which controls the cell's metabolism to replicate itself and form new viruses. Viruses cause many diseases including influenza (single-stranded RNA), herpes (double-stranded DNA), AIDS (a RETROVIRUS, single-stranded RNA) and also mumps, chickenpox and polio.

VISCERA the term for organs within the body cavity, usually the abdominal cavity.

VISION the capacity for sight. Light enters the eye through the cornea and the aqueous humour. Next, it passes through the pupil, lens and vitreous humour to impinge upon the retina. There the ROD and CONE cells detect light and send impulses to the nerve fibres, impulses which are relayed to the visual cortex in the brain. Visual acuity is the sharpness of vision, dependent upon a healthy retina and accurate lens.

VITAMIN any of a group of organic compounds required in very small amounts in the diet to maintain good health. Deficiencies lead to specific diseases. Vitamins are divided into two groups: vitamins A, D, E and K are fat-soluble while C and B are water soluble.

VITREOUS HUMOUR the jelly-like substance occurring between the lens and the retina in the EYE.

VOCAL CORDS two membranes in the LARYNX that vibrate to produce sound when air is expelled over them. Tension in the cords is controlled by muscles and tendons, thus changing the sound generated.

VOLUNTARY MUSCLE (or **STRIATED MUSCLE**) muscle that is under conscious control, e.g. those muscles operating the skeleton. It consists of bundles of elongated fibres surrounded by connective tissue. A

tendon at the end of the muscle attaches it to the bone. Each muscle fibre comprises smaller fibres (*myofibrils*) with alternating dark and light bands (*sarcomeres*), which produce the striated appearance and provide the contractile function. A flexor (or *agonist*) muscle contracts, becoming shorter thus moving bones closer to each other. An extensor or *antagonist* muscle works in the opposite sense.

VOMITING (emesis) the reflex action whereby the stomach contents are expelled through the mouth, due to the contraction of the diaphragm and abdominal wall muscles. Vomiting is due to stimulus of the appropriate centre in the brain but the primary agent is usually a sensation from the stomach itself, e.g. a gastric disease, or some irritant. Other causes may be the action of drugs, some effect on the inner ear (e.g. travel sickness), migraines, etc.

VULVA the external female genitals comprising two pairs of fleshy folds surrounding the vaginal opening.

W

WART (VERRUCA) a solid, benign growth in the skin caused by a virus. They are infectious and spread rapidly in schools, etc. There are several types: *plantar*, on the foot; *juvenile* in children and *venereal*, on the genitals. Warts often disappear spontaneously, but can be dealt with in several ways, e.g. cryosurgery (freezing), laser treatment, and electrocautery (burning away with an electrically heated wire or needle).

WATER ON THE BRAIN see HYDROCEPHALUS.

WEAL (or **WHEAL**) an area of the skin that is temporarily raised and coloured red, or pale with red margins. It may be due to an allergy (*see also* URTICARIA), nettle rash or a sharp blow, and in the former cases may be accompanied by itching.

WEN *see* SEBACEOUS CYST.

WHEEZE the sound produced by the long drawn-out breathing associated with ASTHMA. It also occurs when bronchial tubes are narrowed, e.g. as in BRONCHITIS.

WHIPLASH INJURY damage caused by the sudden jerking backwards of the head and neck, as in a road accident. A severe whiplash can cause death, but injury is the usual outcome. The vertebrae, spinal cord, ligaments and nerves in the neck may all be damaged. Treatment usually involves wearing a special collar to immobilize the affected area.

WHITE MATTER nerve tissue in the CENTRAL NERVOUS SYSTEM, composed primarily of nerve fibres in light-coloured MYELIN sheaths. In the brain it occupies the central part of the cerebral cortex.

WHITLOW inflammation of tissues in the finger tip, and usually an abscess affecting the fat and fibrous tissues that comprise the pulp of the finger.

WHOOPING COUGH (*pertussis*) an infectious disease caused by the bacterium *Bordetella pertussis*. The mucous membranes lining the air passages are affected and after a one to two week incubation period, fever, catarrh and a cough develop. The cough then becomes paroxysmal with a number of short coughs punctuated with the 'whooping' drawing in of breath. Nosebleeds and vomiting may follow a paroxysm. After about two weeks the symptoms abate but a cough may continue for some weeks. Whooping cough is not usually serious and immunization reduces the severity of an attack. However, a child may be susceptible to pneumonia and tuberculosis during the disease.

WINDPIPE *see* TRACHEA.

WISDOM TOOTH the last (third) molar tooth on each side of either jaw. The teeth normally erupt last, around the age of 20 to 25 although some remain impacted in the jaw bone.

WITHDRAWAL SYMPTOMS a characteristic feature when someone stops using a drug upon which they are dependent. Hard drugs such as heroin and cocaine induce dependence as does alcohol, nicotine and amphetamines. Symptoms include shivering, tremors, vomiting and sweating.

WOMB *see* UTERUS.

WOUND a sudden break in the body tissues and/or organs caused by an external agent. There are four types based upon the result of the injury: incisions, punctures, lacerations and contusions.

WRIST the joint between the hand and forearm. The wrist region comprises eight carpal bones and five metacarpal bones joined by strong ligaments. The wrist joint then articulates with the RADIUS and ULNA. The joint can move in all directions with little risk of dislocation.

WRITER'S CRAMP an involuntary contraction of the hand muscles when writing, but not when using those muscles to undertake other functions. A similar condition may arise with musicians (guitarists and pianists), typists and computer operators.

WRYNECK (TORTICOLLIS) when the head is twisted to one side due to a scar contracting or, more commonly, to excessive muscle contraction.

X

X CHROMOSOME the sex chromosome present in male and

female although women have a pair, and men just one (with one Y CHROMOSOME). Certain disorders such as HAEMOPHILIA are carried as genes on the X chromosome.

XIPHOID PROCESS (*or* **XIPHOID CARTILAGE**) the lowest part of the STERNUM. It is a flat cartilage that is progressively replaced by bone, a process completed sometime after middle age.

X-RAYS the part of the electromagnetic spectrum with waves of wavelength 10^{-12} to 10^{-9}m and frequencies of 10^{17} to 10^{21}Hz. They are produced when high velocity electrons strike a target. The rays penetrate solids to a depth that depends upon the density of the solid. X-rays of certain wavelengths will penetrate flesh but not bone. They are therefore useful in therapy and diagnosis within medicine.

Y

Y CHROMOSOME the small chromosome that carries a dominant gene conferring maleness. Normal males have 22 matched chromosome pairs and one unmatched pair comprising one X and one Y chromosome. During sexual reproduction the mother contributes an X chromosome, but the father contributes an X or Y chromosome, XX produces a female offspring, XY male.

Z

ZYGOMATIC ARCH the arch of bone of either side of the face, below the eyes.

ZYGOMATIC BONE a facial bone and one of a pair of bones that form the prominence of the cheeks.

ZYGOTE the cell produced by the fusion of male and female germ cells (GAMETES) during the early stage of fertilization, i.e. an ovum fertilized by a sperm. After passing down the FALLOPIAN TUBE, it implants in the uterus, forming the embryo.